AF341600

IMMUNOLOGICAL PATHOGENESIS OF SEPSIS AND USE OF HEMOSORPTION FOR TREATMENT OF CANCER PATIENTS WITH SEPSIS

Cancer Etiology, Diagnosis and Treatments

Additional books in this series can be found on Nova's website under the Series tab.

Additional e-books in this series can be found on Nova's website under the e-book tab.

IMMUNOLOGICAL PATHOGENESIS OF SEPSIS AND USE OF HEMOSORPTION FOR TREATMENT OF CANCER PATIENTS WITH SEPSIS

NATALIA YU. ANISIMOVA
EDITOR

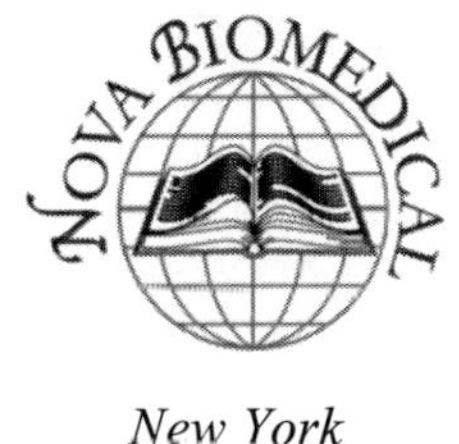

New York

NOTICE TO THE READER

Library of Congress Cataloging-in-Publication Data

ISBN: 978-1-62948-674-1

Library of Congress Control Number: 2013954943

Published by Nova Science Publishers, Inc. † New York

CONTENTS

INTRODUCTION

The monograph is aimed to observe scope and limitations of extracorporeal detoxification, particularly hemosorption, in treatment of cancer patients with sepsis. The topic focused on the research of new approaches and materials for the treatment of patients with generalized infectious complications is appeared to be actual not only for oncology, but for medicine in whole. The data obtained indicate, that in spite of continual improvement of antibacterial therapy, surgery, methods of medicinal correction of cardiovascular and respiratory systems, many patients in postoperative period are faced with systemic inflammatory response syndrome (SIRS), sepsis, severe sepsis, septic shock, which lead to increasing of multiple organ failure and, consequently, often terminated by fatal outcome. Probable reason of insufficient efficiency of current treatment is the limitation of our knowledge about pathogenesis of septic complications. This determines the difficulty in diagnostic before development of clinical presentation, which connected with apparent organ failure. Thus, direct treatment is usually started at the late stage of pathological process, which is the reason of unsuccessful issue. To overcome this barrier it is necessary to reveal the laboratorial criteria, which indicate the initiation of pathological cascade of SIRS, and consequently let to start adequate therapy before clinical presentation. The authors attempted to find out such criteria based on the theory of immunopathogenesis of sepsis. It is known, that septic complications are accompanied with different deep failures of immune system, however, they could be considered as a consequence or as a reason of the development of this pathologic state. Based on the latest suggestion, it is necessary to consider attentively the factors, which initiate the cascade of SIRS (triggers of inflammation), and the biomolecules, which mediate escalation and self-induction of SIRS (mediators of inflammation). The development of the therapeutic approaches, based on these data, seems to be the perspective strategy for the treatment of such dangerous complication as sepsis. Increasing of efficiency of the treatment is supposed to connect with more adequate introduction of the methods of extracorporeal detoxification in therapeutic course of patients with septic complications. However, it is necessary to choose an appropriate method, device and conditions in every particular case.

In: Immunological Pathogenesis of Sepsis … ISBN: 978-1-62948-674-1
Editor: Natalia Yu. Anisimova © 2014 Nova Science Publishers, Inc.

Chapter 1

IMMUNOLOGICAL PATHOGENESIS OF SEPSIS: DIAGNOSTIC AND PROGNOSTIC MARKERS OF SEPSIS

*N. Yu. Anisimova[*], A. Yu. Grebenko, E. G. Gromova,
L. S. Kuznetsova, J. I. Dolzhikova and M. V. Kiselevsky*
N.N. Blokhin Russian Cancer Research Center, Russian Academy
of Medical Sciences, Kashirskoe Sh, 24, 115478, Moscow,
Russian Federation

ABSTRACT

The goal of the study, which was carried out on the basis of N.N. Blokhin Russian Cancer Research Center of RAMS, was to determine the study informativeness of cellular and humoral immunity factors of cancer patients for early diagnosis of septic complications and clinical outcome prognosis. We studied the blood serum of cancer patients admitted to the intensive care unit with severe sepsis and septic shock, cancer patients without any signs of organ failure or multi-organ dysfunction syndrome (MODS) and control group of healthy donors. Our study revealed significant diagnostic indicators associated with sepsis in cancer patients during postoperative period: increase of adhesion molecules expression (CD11b) caused by decrease of apoptosis marker CD95 on the membrane of leukocytes, increase of blood serum factors concentration (IL-6, IL-

---

[*] Corresponding author: Email: n.u.anisimova@gmail.com.

10, IL-18, LPS, sR TNF I, sCD14) and change in the functional activity of leukocytes (NK-activity, phagocytosis) in comparison with the clinical parameters of patients without signs of SIRS. It was also shown that increasing concentrations of IL-8, IL-10 and sR IL-1 II in the blood of patients with sepsis and septic shock are negative prognostic factor, correlated with 28-day mortality of cancer patients.

The choice of disease's effective treatment primarily depends on understanding the causes, mechanisms of development, stage of disease and adequate assessment of the severity of patient's condition. It is especially difficult to do in studying of approaches to the treatment of those diseases, which pathogenesis is still not fully understood. Most of all, it relates to systemic septic complications, which are result of SIRS, proceeding like endotoxicosis in the stage of sub-compensation and decompensation. Meanwhile, in modern oncology, this problem leaves extremely urgent. Immunocompromised condition of cancer patients is caused by a response to the underlying disease and by the need for advanced surgical procedures, prolonged chemo-, radio- and hormone therapy and was associated with increased risk of septic complications in these patients [1-4]. According to obtained data of D.C. Angus, which analyzed statistical data about the mortality of patients in different types of hospitals in several countries, the risk of death from severe sepsis in cancer patients is 30% higher than in non-cancer patients [5].

According to some experts' opinion, the hope for reducing mortality of patients with diagnosed sepsis is the need for improved early diagnostic methods and the use of modern medical technologies, based on the principles of anticipatory etiopathogenetic therapy. Nowadays, the standard measures of intensive therapy of sepsis are early and aggressive antibiotic therapy, which are directed to ensure the hemodynamic stability and metabolism of the patient [6]. Therapeutic approaches, which are aimed at restoring the balance of the immune system, have, unfortunately, only the secondary importance.

The efficacy of appropriate therapy methods increases when they are applied at the early stages of the SIRS, before development of structural disorders in the tissues of vital organs, caused by impacts endo- and exotoxins of microorganisms and autocatalytic processes that is realized in reducing the mortality rate and severity of complications [6-9]. Therefore, the search for early markers that predicted SIRS, sepsis, MODS and outcome of the disease is an extremely important goal of modern medicine in general, and, in particular, oncology. According to modern concepts, the basis of SIRS is dysregulation of immune system of macroorganism, and so, along with the traditionally used criteria such as the PCT, C-reactive protein, increased lactatedehydrogenase, bilirubine, alkaline phosphatases, transaminases, amylase, urea, creatinine, the average molecular weight and some other criteria, there is a promising study of the humoral and cellular parameters of the immune system, and also the level of triggers and mediators of inflammation in the blood serum in order to assess the risk of systemic inflammatory complications in postoperative period patients.

In the described prospective study there were analyzed blood samples of 115 cancer patients, which were admitted to the intensive care unit of N.N. Blokhin Russian Cancer Research Center after extended surgery with the diagnosis of sepsis (n = 22), septic shock (n = 43), acute renal failure (n = 13), acute hepatic failure (n = 8), acute renal failure, following by chronic renal failure (n = 6) and cancer patients without evidence of organ failure (n = 23) and also control group of healthy donors (n = 29).

Recognizing the significant role of pro- and anti-inflammatory cytokines, which are responsible for the integration of key parts of the immune system and intercellular interactions in the escalation of systemic inflammatory process, stimulated the search for reliable markers of inflammation that may be used for diagnosing and prediction of clinical outcome of pathological process. Serum cytokine profile studies of cancer patients and healthy donors revealed that 13 of the examined cytokines (IL-6, IL-8, IL-10, INFγ, TNFα, TNFβ, IL-1β, IL-4, IL-17, IL -2, IL-18, IL-5) of patients with sepsis and septic shock were significantly (p <0.05) revealed increase of concentration of only three: IL-6, IL-10 and IL-18 (Table.1.1). Thus, median IL-6 in the blood of patients with severe sepsis or septic shock was 399 pg/ml and 149 pg/ml against derivation values 25%-75% quartiles from 60 pg/ml to 747 pg/ml, whereas values in the control group were 12 (5-20) pg/ml, and in 25% of healthy donors blood those cytokine was practically not detected. Similarly, the serum concentration of IL-18 in the development of such complications like sepsis and septic shock, increased by several times (1296 (633-2067) pg/ml and 542 (351-1003) pg/ml) in comparison with the control group (163 (123-202) pg/ml). Level of IL-10 showed a less difference: sepsis - 48 (34-128) pg/ml and septic shock - 59 (37-235) pg/ml, and 28 (12-33) pg/ml in the control group. The obtained data corresponds with the conclusions of some researchers, that the increasing level of IL-18 and IL-6 is a characterized indicator of the development of septic complications [10-12]. It is known that these mediators are pleiotropic. In particular, IL-18 is involved in the polarization of T-helper (Th) 1 [13], acting as a stimulation co-factor of Th2 and production of IgE [14] and INF γ by T-cells. It stimulates the release of

IL-2, proliferation and perforin-mediated activity of natural killers [15,16]. IL-6 induces the production of a wide spectrum of acute phase proteins in liver that limits the inflammation. This is, in particular, confirmed by our data, that the content of that cytokine significantly increased not only in acute renal failure, following by sepsis, but also in acute hepatic failure (increased on 200 pg/ml and 186 pg/ml respectively against almost undetectable values in the control group). In septic shock, this cytokine may have a direct damaging effect on the organs and tissues, and, in particular, have a depressing effect on the myocardium [17,18]. This fixed fact of serum blood increased concentration of IL-10 in the prevailing number of patients with septic complications is corresponded with data of prof. A. R. Tuguz, that reported about activation of the expression of mRNA IL-10 in the first hours after surgery (1-3 h) and stabile growth of this cytokine in the blood of cancer patients following by development of SIRS signs, which allowed to conclude about informativity of this value as a marker of postoperative complications [19]. It is interesting that despite the lack of reliably confirmed differences between the cytokine profile of patients with sepsis and septic shock, the latter have a lower level of free cytokines IL-6 and IL-18 and higher level of anti-inflammatory cytokine IL-10 in the blood serum. According to data of our research, an overwhelming number of patients have no difference in level of pro-inflammatory cytokines in comparison with control group, despite the large amount of published data about significant prevalence of their levels during septic complications. This is consistent with data of E. Abraham, that were obtained during multicenter studies, about statistically insignificant efficacy of monoclonal antibodies to IL-1β and TNFα like treatment of patients with sepsis and septic shock [20]. Moreover, blocking IL-1β accompanied by increased mortality of patients. It is worth noting, that, analyzing the levels of other cytokines, some patients reached very high concentrations of IL-8, TNFα and TNFβ during development of complications: 316 pg/ml, 548 pg/ml and 8,900 pg/ml in sepsis, 1243 pg/ml, 548 pg/ml and 1100 pg/ml in septic shock. In healthy donors, the range of deviations of these inflammatory cytokines was significantly shorter: 0-154 pg/ml, 0-17 pg/ml, and 0-38 pg/ml respectively.

To investigate the relationship between serum cytokines and mortality in sepsis, there were analyzed levels of these mediators in the blood serum of survived patients and patients who died within 28 days after taking of blood samples for research. The carried analysis showed no significant difference of serum cytokines (IL-1β, IL-2, IL-4, IL-5, IL-6, IL-12, IL-17, IL-18, INFγ,

TNF α, TNF β) in groups of patients with different clinical outcome. Analysis of the IL-8 and IL-10 concentrations showed a significant difference in content of these mediators in the blood of patients with septic complications, divided into groups according to the measure of 28-day mortality (Figure 1.1).

It should be noted, that, although, the analysis did not reveal significant changes in the content of TNF α and TNF β in the serum of patients, depending on the outcome of the disease, nearly 25% of patients in pre-terminal period have a high content of these mediators (more than 500 pg/ml).

The probable reason of low informativity of serum cytokine profile studies of patients with sepsis is that currently available commercial test systems provide only the concentration measurement of unbound (soluble, free) cytokines. This is a serious obstacle to estimate the total amount of the cytokine induced by the bloodstream. In the absence of free cytokines in the blood there can be their membrane-bound forms or serum receptor-ligand complexes, so-called "hiddencytokinemia" - the presence of high concentrations of cytokines in the biological fluids, which cannot be detected by routine methods [19]. Such hypothesis is supported by reports of several authors about high concentration of some cytokines (IL-6, IL-1β) in the urine and wound discharge on the background of the SIR rise (up to 5000 pg/ml) in cancer patients during the postoperative period [19].

For thorough study of the synthesis of cytokines in patient, we carried out a comparative study of cytokine-induced activity of blood cells before and after stimulation with mitogens. The level of spontaneous production characterizes the initial level of blood cells physiological activity and the intensity of the mitogen-induced production of cytokines that can reveal potential reactivity of blood cells in response to probable antigenic aggression.

The obtained results of our studies indicated that the level of spontaneous production of most analyzed cytokines by blood cells of patients with sepsis did not significantly differ from the values of the control group, and only the spontaneous production of IL-8 in patients with sepsis was 3.5 times higher than the corresponding value of healthy donors (p = 0.044). Mitogen-induced blood cell reactivity in patients with sepsis was reduced, and the level of spontaneous and induced production of basic cytokines was not significantly different, whereas cell stimulation with mitogens in healthy donor led to a significant rise of their concentration in the cultivation medium. It should be noted that, despite the high concentration of serum IL-6 in cancer patients with sepsis, there was observed no significant difference in production of that cytokine by blood cells of patients with complications and healthy donors. The probable cause of high blood level of this pro-inflammatory cytokine is its overproduction by resident macrophages (particularly by Kupffer cells in the liver), which correlates with the synthesis of acute phase proteins [21]. As follows from the obtained data, red blood cells of cancer patients with sepsis, on the background of spontaneous IL-8 overproduction, were often unresponsive to antigenic stimulation, i.e. they were not able to increase the synthesis of cytokines further. This phenomenon can be interpret not only as a manifestation of a reduced reactivity of the effectors' cells, but also as a consequence of inflammatory mediators overproduction on the background of the septic process, which exhausted the secretory potential of innate immunity cells. However, this phenomenon is possibly increased production or shedding from the cell membrane of cytokine receptors that bind free cytokines, which blocks the secondary autocrine synthesis of mediators [19].

Table 1.1. Comparative analysis of cytokine concentrations in the blood serum of cancer patients with severe sepsis, septic shock, patients without infection and normal donors, Median (25%-75%), pg/ml

Cytokines	Groups							p
	Patients with sepsis		Patients with septic shock		Patients without evidence of organ failure		Healthy donors	
IL-1β	0	(0-1)	6	(0-42)	1	(0-5)	16	(0-35)	0. 116
IL-2	43	(37-55)	40	(34-45)	15	(7-42)	16	(5-88)	0,058
IL-4	7	(3-8)	5	(3-13)	17	(15-20)	18	(15-19)	0,11
IL-5	49	(18-88)	69	(22-83)	14	(10-17)	14	(12-19)	0,058
IL-6	399[1,2]	(107-747)	149[1,2]	(60-505)	20	(2-48)	12	(5-20)	0,0001
IL-8	14	(6-57)	22	(7-288)	13	(9-16)	48	(17-140)	0,289
IL-10	48[1,2]	(34-128)	59[1,2]	(37-235)	13	(2-40)	28	(12-33)	0,0001
IL-12	69	(67-95)	56	(46-59)	16	(7-25)	15	(4-28)	0,105
IL-17	65	(0-94)	31	(0-77)	4	(1-9)	30	(15-44)	0,329
IL-18	1296[1,2]	(633-2067)	542[1,2]	(351-1003)	191	(187-200)	163	(123-202)	0,0008
INFγ	0	(0-13)	0	(0-19)	5	(1-13)	5	(2-11)	0,665
TNFα	5	(0-24)	2	(0-19)	0	(0-1)	14	(8-24)	0,057
TNFβ	0	(0-70)	40	(0-150)	11	(3-21)	17	(15-21)	0,643

[1] p<0,05 versus healthy donors.

[2] p<0,05 versus patients without evidence of organ failure.

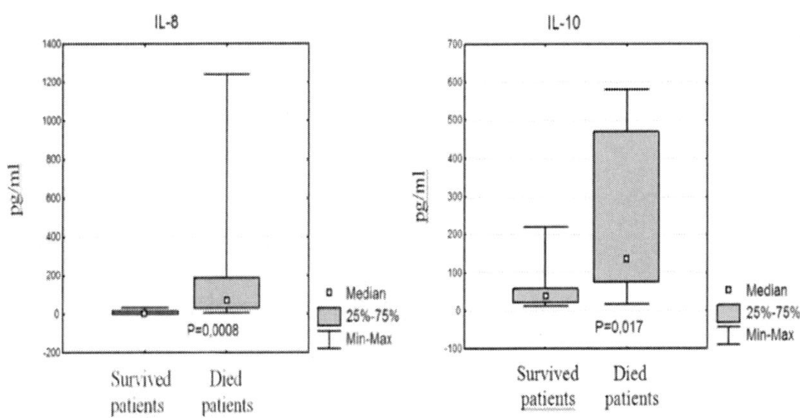

Figure 1.1. Comparative analysis of cytokine level in blood of patients with septic complications, divided into groups according to the measure of 28-day mortality.

Thus, low levels of serum cytokines may not reflect the true concentrations of these mediators in the blood and may be result of not only hyporeactivity of effectors of patients' immunity (as previously thought), but also be the result of specific binding of increased concentrations of soluble receptors. Despite of long-held beliefs about the local (auto-, intra- and paracrine) mechanisms of cytokines action, the existence of undetected, but activated forms of the mediators suggests the possibility of their longer persistence in the systemic circulation. Taking that fact into consideration, it seems appropriate to study not only the cytokines, but also the factors, causing their specific binding in the blood - the soluble cytokine receptors, which are powerful regulators of the activity and level of cytokines, that fix them as firmly as the membrane-bound receptors and protect them from dissolution by blood proteases [22]. In the works of a number of researchers there are data on significant differences of some soluble cytokine receptors serum levels in patients with sepsis: sR TNF RI and sR TNF II [19,23], sR IL-1 II [24] and sR IL-6 [25-27].

According to the results of our researches (demonstrated in Table 1.2) only serum level of sR TNF I (p55) was significantly increased in the blood of cancer patients with sepsis (in 5-6 times in comparison with healthy donors), while statistical significance of sR IL-1 II and s R IL-6 as markers of sepsis was not confirmed.

Table1.2. Comparative analysis of cytokine receptors concentrations in the blood serum of cancer patients with severe sepsis, septic shock, patients without infection and normal donors, Median (25%-75%), pg/ml

Analytes	Groups								p
	Patients with sepsis		Patients with septic shock		Patients without evidence of organ failure		Healthy donors		
sR TNF I	78 [1,2]	(53-248)	60 [1]	(50-96)	15	(11-30)	12	(10-19)	*0,0001*
sR IL-1II	3853	(2407-5505)	382	(267-3337)	2003	(354-2564)	2564	(2387-2789)	*0,195*
sR IL-6	52300	(4752-54100)	49900	(37320-53560)	10784	(2386-22415)	44322	(10897-46998)	*0,074*

[1] p<0,05 versus healthy donors.

[2] p<0,05 versus patients without evidence of organ failure.

Table 1.3. Comparative analysis of LPS and LPS-associated peptides in the blood serum of cancer patients with severe sepsis, septic shock, patients without infection and normal donors, Median (25%-75%), pg/ml

Analytes	Patients with sepsis		Patients with septic shock		Patients without evidence of organ failure		Healthy donors		p
LPS, U/ml	1.5 [1,2]	(0,48-5,5)	1.95 [1,2]	(0,60-3,0)	0.005	(0-0,03)	0	(0-0,001)	*0,0001*
LBP, μg/ml	9	(6,1-11,9)	10.0	(6,8-12,0)	7.0	(5,0-9,0)	8,9	(7,3-10,5)	*0,166*
s CD14, μg/ml	9,9 [1,2]	(8,4-11,8)	12,7 [1,2]	(7,1-13,0)	2,8	(2,1-4,6)	3,4	(1,7-3,7)	*0,0004*

[1] p<0,05 versus healthy donors.

[2] p<0,05 versus patients without evidence of organ failure.

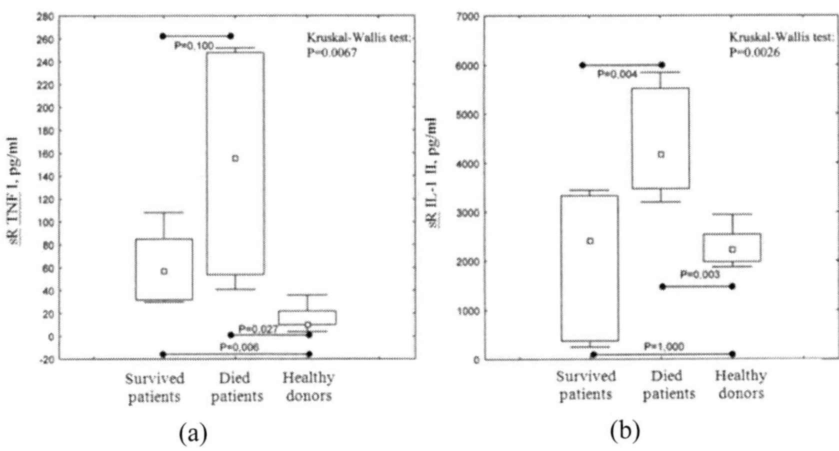

Figure 1.2. Comparative analysis of cytokine receptors level in blood of patients with septic complications, divided into groups according to the measure of 28-day mortality.

However, the level of sR IL-1 II was significantly higher in the blood of patients who died 4176 (3475-5526) pg/ml compared with the survived patients - 2407 (374-3334) pg/ml and healthy donors - 2564 (2387-2789) pg/ml (Figure 1.2). The significant difference in the level of the receptors in the blood serum of cancer patients without symptoms of septic complications and control groups was not detected. According to the available data in the references [28], the cause of concentration increase of soluble receptors, along with the shedding of membrane-bound forms, is de novo enhanced synthesis of alternatively spliced mRNA, which is directly associated with increased production of corresponding cytokine. Therefore, the established fact of serum concentrations increase of the receptor may indicate hypercytokinemia [29]. This assumption is confirmed by correlation analysis, conducted in our study, that allowed us to establish a close correlation (p<0.05) between the level of sR TNF I and the blood serum level of cytokines TNFβ, TNFα, IL-8, IL-6, which may indicate a hidden hypercytokinemia of tumor factor necrosis and IL-8 in cancer patients with sepsis. The fact that from the 3 tested receptors to cytokines there was significantly increased only one sR TNF I, may be explained by the increased synthesis of TNF that can be positively correlated with the production of not only sR TNF I, but also sR TNF II, which does not participate in the transduction of the signal from the receptor, but, however, bind it, acting as a "mediator trap". It was found by prof. A.R. Tuguz, that 1ml of blood produced sR TNF II in much larger quantities than sR TNF I [30]. It should be noted that R TNF I is an "domain of death" – it is receptor that transduces a signal to apoptosis and its increased shedding from cell membranes, its transfromation to a serum soluble form means reduction of cells sensitivity to the signals of apoptosis initiation.

The study of serum levels of other receptors to cytokines may be important for identification of prediction factors of disease development. We found that concentration increase of sR IL-1 II, along with IL-8, IL-10 in the blood serum is associated with an increased risk of an adverse clinical outcome, because it is directly correlated with the criteria of 28-day mortality.

Thus, our data reflect the trend growth of uncontrolled cytokines overexpression in the development of septic processes, which called "cytokine storm". The reason for this phenomenon may be the increase of cytokine-induced cells and production of mediators due to hyperactive state of effectors. There is significant increase in the leukocytes concentration, both in sepsis and septic shock, mainly due to neutrophilia.

In our study of patients in septic shock, there was observed more remarkably left shift than in patients with sepsis, by increasing the number of band neutrophils. On the background of neutrophilia we noticed a relative reduction of lymphocytes in the blood serum, but the absolute number of these cells remained within the physiological range: sepsis - 1,5 (1,3-3) $\times$ 10^9 cells/ml and septic shock 1.9 (1,5-2,2) $\times$ 10^9 cells/ml.

It is interesting that leukocytes (CD45+cells) in blood of patients with sepsis had a significant expression increase of adhesion molecules CD11b compared with healthy donors. There was marked a significant increase in both absolute and relative number of CD45+ CD11b+ effectors (Figure 1.3.).

Similarly, the unambiguous trend of enhanced expression on leukocytes CD11a and CD11c, which is associated with an increase of the activation degree of immunocompetent cells [31], because it is known that the membrane concentration of CD11b correlated with the ability to polymerize actin (the main component of cytoskeleton[32]), and CD11c correlated with implementation of the complement-depended phagocytosis. In addition, transendothelial emigration of granulocytes in tissue is powered by β2 integrins such as CD11b (CR3 or Mac1). Due to increase of their expression, it is likely to be fatal change in the functional activity of immune effector cells in sepsis. Also, it should be noted, that the high level of presentation of these adhesion molecules on the cell membrane may cause disorders of blood rheological properties, as they bind neutrophils and macrophages on the endothelium and migrate into the tissues.

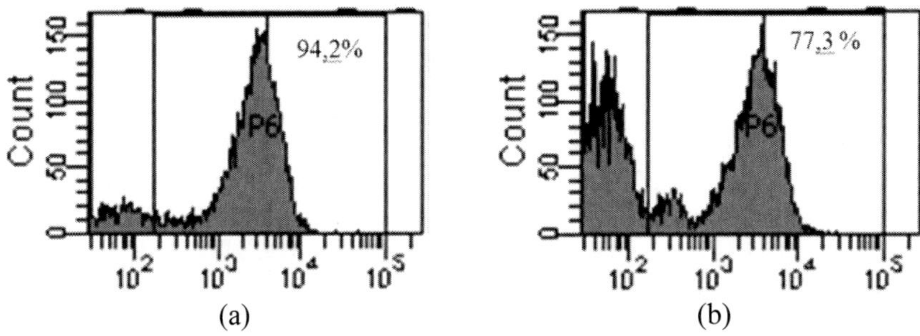

(a)   (b)

Figure 1.3. The increase of relative number of CD45+ CD11b+ leukocytes in blood of cancer patients with sepsis (a) in comparison with healthy donors (b).

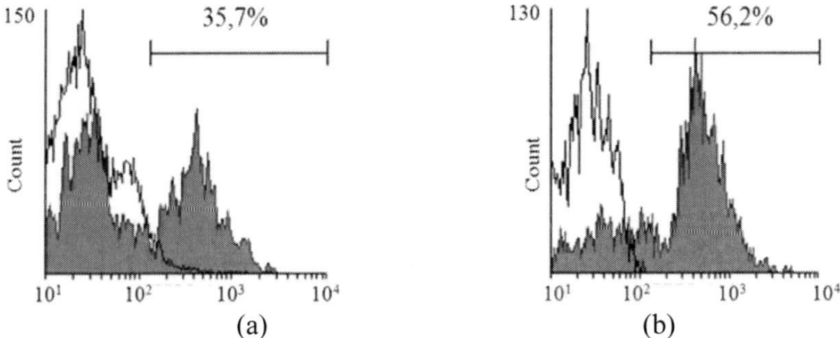

(a)   (b)

Figure 1.4. The decrease of relative number of CD45+ CD95+ leukocytes in blood of cancer patients with sepsis (a) in comparison with healthy donors (b).

Immunosuppression state, which is usually associated with increased risk of systemic inflammation in patients with sepsis caused by apoptosis of immunocompetent cells. A number of researchers noted an increase in the expression of apoptosis receptor CD95 (Fas) on T-cells of patients in the postoperative period [33] and considered this phenomenon as an indication of a developing lymphopenia. However, according to our data, there is marked decrease of subpopulations CD45+ CD95+ cells in the blood of patients with sepsis, on the background of a significant increase of their absolute number in the systemic circulation (Figure1.4).

A similar trend was observed for populations of neutrophils and monocytes, which carry over domain, responsible for apoptosis signal on their membrane. Similar results were obtained by other researchers [34-37], which correlated with the provisions about intense shedding of "domain of death" sR TNF I, which also prevented apoptosis, making the cell resistant to the signal.

There is evidence, that the level decrease of CD95 expression on neutrophils is correlated with the severity of the inflammatory process [38]. It was found that increasing the life of leukocyte cells can lead to damage of tissues and organs in SIRS and sepsis [39,40], and so changes in the regulation of apoptosis as the process, that is responsible for removal of senescent cells from the body plays an crucial role in the pathogenesis of sepsis and multiple organ failure [41]. Lymphopenia is the reason of hyporeactivity of immune system in sepsis. According to our data, on the background of decrease trend of the relative number of lymphocytes and some subpopulations (T-helper cells and NK-cells), the absolute content of these cells in the bloodstream correspond or exceed those in healthy donors. However, according to our data, the index of CD4/CD8 in sepsis patients was significantly lower (0.03-0.06) than in healthy donors (1.1-2.2), which may indicate an balance disorder of Th1 and Th2 lymphocytes with a prevalence of Th2 cells in the circulating blood, or a long persistence of Th2 cells in the blood as a result of the apoptosis signaling system loss. In any case, the result of such imbalance is a significant change in the synthesis, induction and persistence of the pro- and anti-inflammatory cytokines in the blood that reflects in change of serum cytokine profile. The results of concentrations rise of inflammatory mediators in blood may be sigh of hyperactivation of immune effector cells, their induction of aggressive tissue-damaging factors, and especially the endothelium-damaging factors, the development of organ failure and multiple organ failure with high mortality risk.

Large amounts of bacterial toxins release into the blood and circulate in the bloodstream. They coact with inflammatory mediators and activate cells. Wehave found that level of bacterial endotoxin in the blood serum of patients with sepsis and septic shock was significantly increased: sepsis - 1.5 (0,48-5,5) U/ml, septic shock - 1.95 (0,6-3,0) U/ml compared with patients without postoperative complications - 0,005 (0-0,03) U/ml and healthy donors - 0 (0-0,001) U/ml (Table 1.3).

This analyte was detected in the blood of 73-75% of patients with developed postoperative septic complications - that may indicate that the source of infection was not the pathogens from the primary focus, but the natural flora of the body's mucous membranes, primarily intestine. It can emerge in the blood due to decreased barrier function. The reasons can be surgical stress and high-dose antibiotic therapy [42,43]. The basic cellular mechanism of bacterial translocation is transcytosis of bacteria by specialized M-cells of the intestinal epithelium. It was found in the middle of 90's of XX century [44]. The peculiarity of the M-cells is that they capture and transport different antigens (bacteria, microparticles) from the intestinal lumen to the lymphoid tissue - that is the function of transintestinal antigen transport, which significance remains unknown.

LBP, along with the soluble receptor CD14, is transport system for LPS, and many researchers consider these proteins as potential markers of endotoxemia and development of septic complications. However, the results of our study didn't confirm the fact of significant LBP level increase in sepsis, opposed to existing literature data, although there was set a trend to its increase in the blood in sepsis (Table 1.3). Significant individual variations of that parameter in sepsis and septic shock were noted (1-19,7mkg/ml and 0,7-21,8 mkg/ml, respectively). At the same time, LBP level of more than 25% of patients exceeds the maximum values which were recorded in healthy donors and patients without complications (12 µg/ml). There were obtained interesting data in a comparative analysis of serum LPS and LBP levels in the groups of survived and died patients with sepsis. In particular, in the blood of patients with a poor prognosis there were showed much higher level of LPS, which indicate the loss of the mucous barrier function and enhancing the potential translocation of pathogenic microflora into the internal environment of the body. There was observed a significant decrease in the level of specific binding protein (LBP) of this group of patients. This may be due to the depletion of the serum protein fraction because of binding by LPS excess, and due to the synthesis decrease of LBP in hepatocytes. As a result, there was decrease correlation of serum LBP level with poor outcome in cancer patients with sepsis, that accompanied by LBP/LPS reduction in about 10 times, compared with the survived patients.

Comparative analysis of sCD14 serum concentration revealed significant differences between patients with septic complications and donors: the concentration of that analyte in sepsis was 2.9 times, and in septic shock - 3.7 times higher than in healthy donors (Table 1.3). There were no significant differences between patients with sepsis or septic shock, as well as between patients without septic complications and healthy donors. The foregoing suggests that the concentration increase of LPS and sCD14, on the background of simultaneous lowering of LBP in the blood, should be regarded as a poor prognostic sign in cancer patients with sepsis.

Table 1.4. Comparative analysis of serum level of immunoglobulins in the blood of cancer patients with severe sepsis, septic shock, patients without infection and normal donors, Median (25%-75%), pg/ml

Analytes	Groups								p
	Patients with sepsis		Patients with septic shock		Patients without evidence of organ failure		Healthy donors		
IgA, µg/ml	1,74	(0,85-2,36)	1,78	(0,83-2,41)	1,65	(1,10-2,20)	2,30	(1,30-2,45)	0,638
Ig M, µg/ml	0,75	(0,34-1,77)	0,75	(0,41-1,89)	1,55	(1,05-1,90)	2,22	(1,42-2,32)	0,05
Ig G, µg/ml	10,05	(6,57-15,91)	13,20	(8,11-15,78)	10,00	(9,50-10,20)	11,37	(10,62-11,66)	0,465

Table 1.5. The parameters of the phagocytic activity of cancer patients with sepsis and patients without infection with sepsis compared with healthy donors, Median (25%-75%)

Parameters	Stimulatorsofphagocytosis	Healthy donors (control)	Cancer patients	
			without infection	with sepsis
Index of phagocytosis , %	latex	28 (21-33)	30 (20-46)	76* (72-97)
	yeast	15 (9-27)	-	52* (41-62)
	L. acidophilus	21 (12-25)	-	62* (31-57)
Phagocytic number, equivalent units	latex	6 (3-7)	7 (5-15)	38* (29-52)
	yeast	1 (1-2)	-	5* (4-8)
	L. acidophilus	1 (1-1)	-	4* (3-7)
Basic NBT test, equivalent units		0,15 (0,09÷0,32)	0,52 (0,28÷0,70)	2,35* (1,90÷2,50)
NBT test induced by latex, equivalent units		1,20** (1,10÷1,31)	1,41** (1,28÷1,60)	2,50* (2,20÷2,81)

* - p<0.05 versus control.

** - p<0.05, induced NBT test versus basic NBT test.

As the data above indicate that the activation of immunocompetent cells play an important role in the development of SIRS, we can assume that the secondary immune response is directed to the elimination of intracellular and extracellular pathogens and is determined by the activity of B-cells, mediated by immunoglobulins and it will also undergo significant changes. Bacterial lipopolysaccharidies are capable of polyclonal activation of large populations of B-lymphocytes at a sufficiently high concentration. However, there are some reports of significant level decrease of different classes of antibodies on the background of development of sepsis signs, so that some researchers postulate the importance of reducing some subclasses of immunoglobulins as markers of sepsis.

According to the results of our studies (demonstrated in Table 1.4), there are no statistically significant differences were detected between the serum concentrations of Ig M, Ig A, Ig G between groups of cancer patients with septic complications, patients with no complications and healthy donors (p = 0.05). However, there is detected trend to decrease concentration of Ig M in sepsis and septic shock on the background of significant variation of initial values (both above extreme values of the control group and those below). This result is consistent with the fact that there was no observed signs of significant subpopulation reduction of CD45+CD3-CD19+ cells (B-lymphocytes) in blood: 1.2 (0.6-1.8%) in sepsis patients and 2.1 (1,0-2,3%) in healthy donors.

The absence of proteins depletion of these fractions does not change the application value of exogenous immunoglobulin for treatment patients with sepsis, because, as it is known, the role of antibodies in the development of postoperative complications are obviously not only binding, segregation and degradation of antigenic substances. There are antigen-associated immune-globulins that have a number of regulatory functions. Thus, there is detected, antigen-specific, dependent on activated T-lymphocytes and complement, increased in 50-100 times immune response by corpuscular or soluble antigen complexes with IgM-antibodies[45]. In addition, administration of immune-globulin preparations can have a normalizing effect on restoring the activity balance of Th1 and Th2 lymphocytes populations.

As mentioned above, there is significant amount of bacterial toxins in the blood in septic complications, especially LPS and such cytokines like IL- 10, IL- 6, IL- 18. Therefore, first of all, it is reasonable to expect a significant change in the functional activity of the effectors of innate immunity (NK-cells, granulocytes and monocytes), which play a crucial role in the pathogenesis of sepsis [46]. The peculiarities of innate immune effectors response to the microbial pathogen play a special role in the development of the SIRS, which is linked with inflammation as a typical adaptive response, but in certain conditions it can be pathological.

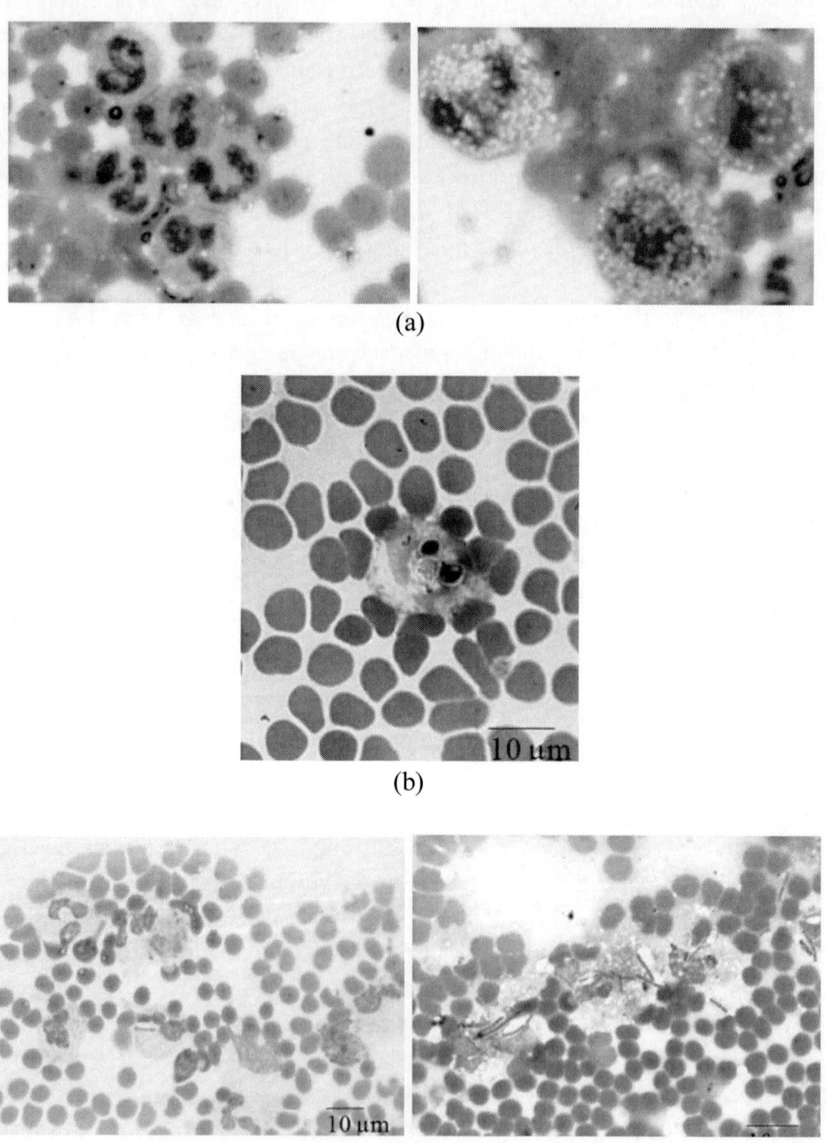

Figure 1.5. The neutrophils of cancer patient without signs of inflammatory (left) and cancer patients with sepsis (right) after incubation (t = 40 min) with the latex beads (a), yeast (b) and L. acidophilus (c).

In our study we found a significant activity of NK in blood in cancer patients with sepsis (up to 39%) in comparison with healthy donors and patients without complications. These data are consistent with the results of other authors, which previously reported about increased level of NK activity in patients with septic postoperative complications [47]. There is data in the literature, that this phenomenon, in particular, can be mediated by the effects of IL-12 on immune cells of the blood that enhanced the cytotoxicity of NK-cells and T-killer cells and induction of granzymes A and B which are the effector molecules that mediate the cytotoxicity [47]. We noticed a trend of increasing concentration of this cytokine in the systemic circulation, as in sepsis and septic shock, although the statistical significance of this fact was questionable ($p > 0.05$) (Table 1.1). However, from our point of view, the most likely explanation for this phenomenon was significant 1,5 times increase in the proportion of CD45+ CD3- CD16 + CD56+ cells, identified as natural killers in the lymphocyte populations of the blood, that resulted in a significant increase in the cytotoxic activity of ML blood of patients with sepsis (at 1.2-2.2 times higher than in control group) in vitro. Thus, there were detected no statistically significant difference in NK-activity values of healthy donors and patients with malignant neoplasms without complications ($p > 0.05$).

Furthermore, there were obtained data about significant intensity increase of the phagocytic activity of granulocytes (Table 1.4, Fig. 1.5).

This phenomenon was studied after stimulation of leukocytes by latex and microorganisms (by bacteria andunicellular fungi). That was needed to study the reactivity of neutrophils in the presence of agents of various types that initiate phagocytosis. There was measured phagocytic index - the number of cells, that was able to capture foreign particles or cells and phagocytic number, that allows to assess the potential of its internalization by the phagocyte. The number of active phagocytes (the index of phagocytosis or the phagocytic index -PI) in patients with sepsis after stimulation with latex was increased almost threefold compared with healthy donors (median values corresponded to 76% and 28%), and the intensity of the particle capture by a single phagocyte (phagocytic number -PN) increased by 6.3 times (38 and 6 units, respectively). It was noted, that the ability of blood neutrophils of patients with sepsis to phagocytosis of gram-positive bacteria was significantly increased (PI of patients was threefold higher in comparison with donors) and also number of granulocytes, capable to the yeasts' internalisation, was 3.5-fold increased. The intensity of the absorption of phagocyte microorganisms also increased significantly more than 4-fold after stimulation by bacteria and 5-fold after stimulation by yeasts. This is due to a significant proportion increase of leukocytes in the blood of cancer patients with sepsis, that express adhesion molecule on the membrane (CD11a, CD11b and CD11c), providing close contact with phagocytised objects and thus involved in the implementation of phagocytosis. Perhaps, increased production of pro-inflammatory cytokines by immunocompetent cells of blood (in particular, IL-8 - a key cytokine, that take part in the recruitment of neutrophils to the site of inflammation and stimulate their activity) caused the activation of neutrophils. The functional activity of neutrophils of cancer patients without complications was similar in comparison with the donors.

CONCLUSION

The data research generalization of serum content informativity of a wide variety of humoral immunity mediators and LPS for the diagnosis of systemic suppurative inflammatory conditions that developed in the postoperative period in cancer patients let us to make a conclusion about inexpediency of carrying out such a laborious research. In particular, the study of profile and production of wide spectrum of cytokines by immunocompetent cells may be limited and there will be needed to determinate levels of IL-6, IL-10, IL-8, IL-18 and congruent receptors - sR TNF I and sCD14, which concentrations are significantly higher than those of healthy donors. It may be considered as markers of sepsis and septic shock in cancer patients. Of course, there was highly informative study of LPS level in the blood. Furthermore, in order to predict the severity of SIRS, there should be recognized informative to determinate IL-8, IL-10 and sR IL-1 II levels in a blood serum of patients with suppurative septic complications. However, it should be noted that during our study, the concentration increase of any of these analytes are not 100% correlated with clinical signs of manifestation of SIRS symptoms, i.e. informativity of these parameters ranged from 75% (cytokines and their receptors) to 88 % (LPS). At the same time, the study of functional activity parameters of immunocompetent cells in cancer patients showed high informativity of their assessment, as there was observed a significant increase of the NK-activity and phagocytic activity of neutrophils of less than 91% of patients with sepsis.

REFERENCES

[1] Angus, DC; Linde-Zwirble, WT; Lidicker, J; Clermont, G; Carcillo, J; Pinsky, MR. Epidemiology of severe sepsis in the United States: analysis of incidence, outcome, and associated costs of care. *Crit. Care Med.*, 2001, 29, 1303– 1310.

[2] Danai, PA; Sinha, S; Moss, M; Haber, MJ; Martin, GS. Seasonal variation in the epidemiology of sepsis. *Crit .Care Med.*, 2007, 35(2), 410– 415.

[3] Hodgin, KE; Moss, M. The epidemiology of sepsis. *Curr. Pharm. Des.*, 2008, 14(19), 1833– 1839.

[4] Padkin, A; Goldfrad, C; Brady, AR; Young, D; Black, N; Rowan, K. Epidemiology of severe sepsis occurring in the first 24 hrs in intensive care units in England, Wales, and Northern Ireland. *Crit. Care Med.*, 2003, 31(9), 2332– 2338.

[5] Angus, DC; Wax, RS. Epidemiology of sepsis: an update. *Crit. Care Med.*, 2001, 29, S109-S116.

[6] Dellinger, RP; Levy, MM; Carlet, JM; Bion, J; Parker MM; Jaeschke, R; Reinhart, K; Angus, DC; Brun-Buisson, C; Beale, R; Calandra, T., Dhainaut, JF; Gerlach, H; Harvey, M; Marini, JJ; Marshall, J; Ranieri, M; Ramsay, G; Sevransky, J; Thompson, BT; Townsend, S; Vender, JS; Zimmerman, JL; Vincent, JL. Surviving Sepsis Campaign: international guidelines for management of severe sepsis and septic shock. *Intensive Care Med.*, 2008, 34, 17–60.

[7] Foland, JA; Fortenberry, JD; Warshaw, BL; Pettignano, R; Merritt, RK; Heard, ML; Rogers, K; Reid, C; Tanner, AJ; Easley, KA. Fluid overload before continuous hemofiltration and survival in critically ill children: A retrospective analysis. *Crit. Care Med.*, 2004, 32, 1771– 1776.

[8] Peng, ZY; Wang, H; Carter, MJ; DiLeo, M; Kellum, JA. Hemo-adsorption improves long-term survival after sepsis in the rat. *Crit. Care Med.*, 2008, 36 (12 suppl.), A1.

[9] Rivers, EP. Early goal-directed therapy in severe sepsis and septic shock: converting science to reality. *Chest*, 2006, 129(2), 217– 218.

[10] Barber, MD; Fearon, KC; Ross, JA. Relationship of serum levels of interleukin-6, soluble interleukin-6 receptor and tumour necrosis factor receptors to the acute-phase protein response in advanced pancreatic cancer. *Clin. Sci.* (Lond.), 1999, 96(1), 83– 87.

[11] Gaïni, S; Koldkjaer, OG; Pedersen, C; Pedersen, SS. Procalcitonin, lipopolysaccharide-binding protein, interleukin-6 and C-reactive protein in community-acquired infections and sepsis: a prospective study. *Crit. Care.Med.*, 2006, 10 (2), R53.

[12] Grobmyer, SR; Lin, E; Lowry, SF; Rivadeneira, DE; Potter, S; Barieand, PS; Nathan, CF. Elevation of IL-18 in Human Sepsis. *J. ClinImmunol.*, 2000, 20(3), 212– 215.

[13] Dinarello, CA. Interleukin-18 and the pathogenesis of inflammatory diseases. *Semin. Nephrol.*, 2007, 27, 98 – 114.

[14] Dinarello, CA. Immunological and inflammatory functions of the interleukin-1 family. *Ann. Rev. Immunol.*, 2009, 27, 519 – 550.

[15] French, AR; Holroyd, EB; Yang, L; Kim, S; Yokoyama, WM. IL-18 acts synergistically with IL-15 in stimulating natural killer cell proliferation. *Cytokine*, 2006, 35 (5 – 6), 229 – 234.

[16] Hyodo, Y; Matsui, K; Hayashi, N; Tsutsui, H; Kashiwamura, S-i; Yamauchi, H; Hiroishi, K; Takeda, K; Tagawa, Y-I; Iwakura, Y; Kayagaki, N; Kurimoto, M; Okamura, H; Hada, T; Yagita, H; Akira, S; Nakanishi, K; Higashino, K. IL-18 Up-Regulates Perforin-Mediated NK Activity Without Increasing Perforin Messenger RNA Expression by Binding to Constitutively Expressed IL-18 Receptor. *J. Immunol.*, 1999, 162, 1662 – 1668.

[17] Anderson, R; Schmidt, R. Clinical biomarkers in sepsis. *Front Biosci (Elite Ed)*, 2010, 1(2), 504 – 520.

[18] Pinsky, MR. Pathophysiology of sepsis and multiple organ failure:pro- versus anti-inflammatory aspects . *Contrib. Nephrol.*, 2004, 144, 31 – 43.

[19] Tuguz, AR. The imunopatogenesis early postoperative complications in patients with cancer. *Dr. Sci. Thesis*, Moscow, 2002.

[20] Abraham, E; Laterre, PF; Garbino, J; Pingleton, S; Butler,T; Dugernier, T; Margolis, B; Kudsk, K; Zimmerli, W; Anderson, P; Reynaert, M; Lew, D; Lesslauer, W; Passe, S; Cooper, P; Burdeska, A; Modi, M; Leighton, A; Salgo, M; Van der AP. Lenercept (p55 tumor necrosis factor receptor fusion protein) in severe sepsis and early septic shock: a randomized, double-blind, placebo-controlled, multicenter phase III trial with 1342 patients. *Crit. Care Med.*, 2001, 29, 503 – 510.

[21] Jean-Baptiste, E. Cellular Mechanisms in Sepsis. *J. Intensive Care. Med.*, 2007, 22(2), 63 – 72.

[22] Rose-John, S; Heinrich, P. Soluble receptors for cytokines and growth factors: generation and biological function. *Biochem J.*, 1994, 1 300(Pt. 2), 281–90.

[23] Zhang, B; Huang, Y H; Chen, Y; Yang, Y; Hao, Z L; Xie, SL. Plasma tumor necrosis factor-α, its soluble receptors and interleukin-1β levels in critically burned patients. *Burns*, 1998, 24 (7), 599 – 603.

[24] Müller, B; Peri, G; Doni, A; Perruchoud, AP; Landmann, R; Pasqualini, F; Mantovan, A. High circulating levels of the IL-1 type II decoy receptor in critically ill patients with sepsis: association of high decoy receptor levels with glucocorticoid administration. *J. Leuk. Biol.*, 2002, 72, 643 – 649.

[25] Barber, MD; Fearon, KC; Ross, JA. Relationship of serum levels of interleukin-6, soluble interleukin-6 receptor and tumour necrosis factor receptors to the acute-phase protein response in advanced pancreatic cancer. *Clin. Sci.* (Lond.), 1999, 96(1), 83 – 87.

[26] Frieling, JTM; Van Deuren, M; Wijdenes, J; van der Meer, JW; Clement, C; van der Linden, CJ; Sauerwein, RW. Circulating interleukin-6 receptor in patients with sepsis syndrome. *J. Infect. Dis.*, 1995, 171, 469 – 472.

[27] Zeni, F; Tardy, B; Vindimian, M; Pain, P; Gery, P; Bertrand, JC. Soluble interleukin-6 receptor in patients with severe sepsis. *J. Infect. Dis.*, 1995, 172(2), 607 – 608.

[28] Rose-John, S; Heinrich, P. Soluble receptors for cytokines and growth factors: generation and biological function. *Biochem J.*, 1994, 1 300(Pt. 2), 281 – 290.

[29] Gon, KC; Hashimoto, S; Hayashi, S; Koura, T; Matsumoto, K; Horie, T. Lower serum concentrations of cytokines in elderly patients with pneumonia and the impaired production of cytokines by peripheral blood monocytes in the elderly. *Clin. Exp. Immunol.*, 1996, 106(1), 120 – 126.

[30] Anisimova, NYu; Tuguz, AR; Chikileva, IV; Kiselevsky, MV; Golubev IN; Vershinina, MYu; Vorobyev, AA.The influence of possible mechanisms of an increased content of soluble receptors of cytokines sIL-4R, sIL-6R, sTNF-RI, sTNF-Rll in the blood of healthy donors and oncology patients (Russian). *Immunology*, 2003, 2 №2, 113 – 116.

[31] Bhupinder, S M; Kian, FC. Blood neutrophil activation markers in severe asthma: lack of inhibition by prednisolone therapy. *Respiratory Research*, 2006, 7, 59.

[32] Brom, J; Köller, M; Schlüter, B; Müller-Lange, P; Ulrich, H; König, W. Expression of the adhesion molecule CD11b and polymerization of actin by polymorphonuclear granulocytes of patients endangered by sepsis. *Burns*, 1995, 21 (6), 427 – 443.

[33] Delogu, G; Moretti, S; Antonucci, A; Marcellini, S; Masciangelo, R; Famularo, G; Signore, L; De Simone, C. Apoptosis and surgical trauma: dysregulated expression of death and survival factors on peripheral lymphocytes. *Arch. Surg.*, 2000, 135, 1141 – 1147.

[34] Härter, L; Mica, L; Stocker, R; Trentz, O; Keel, M. Mcl-1 correlates with reduced apoptosis in neutrophils from patients with sepsis. *J. Am. Coll. Surg.*, 2003, 197, 964 – 973.

[35] Jimenez, MF; Watson, WG; Parodo, J; Evans, D; Foster, D; Steinberg, M; Rotstein, OD, Marshall, JC. Dysregulated expression of neutrophil apoptosis in the systemic inflammatory response syndrome. *Arch. Surg.*, 1997, 132, 1263 – 1270.

[36] Papathanassoglou, EDE; Moynihan, JA; McDermott, MP; Ackerman, MH. Expression of Fas (CD95) and Fas ligand on peripheral blood mononuclear cells in critical illness and association with multiorgan dysfunction severity and survival. *Crit Care Med.*, 2001, 29, 709 – 718.

[37] Sayeed, MM. Delay of neutrophil apoptosis can exacerbate inflammation in sepsis patients: cellular mechanisms. *Crit. Care Med.*, 2004, 32, 1604 – 1606.

[38] Fialkow, L; Filho, LF; Bozzetti, MC; Milani, AR; Filho, EMR; Ladniuk, RM; Pierozan, P; de Moura, RM; Prolla, JC; Vachon, E; Downey, GP. Neutrophil apoptosis: a marker of disease severity in sepsis and sepsis-induced acute respiratory distress syndrome. *Crit. Care Med.*, 2006, 10(6), R155.

[39] Steven, HW. To die or not to die: an overview of apoptosis and its role in disease. *JAMA*, 1998, 279, 300 – 307.

[40] Ware, LB; Matthay, MA. Clinical progress: the acute respiratory distress syndrome. *N. Engl. J. Med.*, 2000, 342,1334 – 1349.

[41] Mahidhara, R; Billiar, TR. Apoptosis in sepsis. *Crit Care Med.*, 2000, 28, N105 – N113.

[42] Balzan, S; Quadros, CDA; Cleva, RD; Zilberstein, B; Cecconello, I. Bacterial translocation: Overview of mechanisms and clinical impact. *J. Gastroenterol. Hepatol.*, 2007, 22 (4), 464 – 471.

[43] Deitch, A; Bridges, RM. Effect of stress and trauma on bacterial translocation from the gut. *J. Surg Res.*, 1987, 42 (5), 536 – 542.

[44] Neutra, MR. Role of M cells in transepithelial transport of antigens and pathogens to the mucosal immune system. *Am. J. Physiol.*, 1998, 274 (5), G785 – G791.

[45] Klimovich, VB; Samoilovich, MP. Immunoglobulin A (IgA) and its receptors (Russian). *Med. Immunol.*, 2006, 8 № 4, 483 – 500.

[46] Zeerleder, S; Hack, CE; Caliezi, C; van Mierlo, G; Eerenberg-Belmer, A; Wolbink, A; Wuillenmin, WA. Activated cytotoxic T cells and NK cells in severe sepsis and septic shock and their role in multiple organ dysfunction. *ClinImmunol*, 2005, 116(2), 158-65.

[47] Giamarellos-Bourboulis, E J; Tsaganos, T; Spyridaki, E; Mouktaroudi , M; Plachouras, D; Vaki, I; Karagianni, V; Antonopoulou, A; Veloni , V; Giamarellou, H. Early changes of CD4-positive lymphocytes and NK cells in patients with severe Gram-negative sepsis. *Crit Care*, 2006, 10, R166.

Chapter 2

PATHOMORPHOLOGY OF SEPSIS

O. V. Lebedinskay[1] and A. N. Kopylov[2]*
[1]E.A. Vagner Perm Medical Academy, Department of Histology,
Embryology and Cytology, Perm, Russia
[2]N.N. Blokhin Russian Cancer Research Center, RAMS,
Laboratory of Cell Immunity, Moscow, Russia

ABSTRACT

Pathoanatomical research is important for postmortal proof of
clinically-diagnosed sepsis and requires a detailed description of damaged
organs. Also it should be noted that there is no match between
histological data and degrees of organ dysfunctions in septic patients.
Death of cells from the heart, kidneys, lungs, and tissues may be
inconspicuous and perhaps will not show clinical signs of organ
dysfunction. In our research we made an attempt to reveal pathomorphologic features of damage in organs after sepsis in cancer patients.
However we did not observe any particular pathomorphological changes
in organs from patients with complications caused by sepsis. All changes
had pathomorphological signs of multi-organ failure. So pathomorphological changes in organs during sepsis that complicated cancer disease
have no special signs. Special experiments in vivo were performed to
prove pathogenetic influence of microorganism toxins, especially LPS in
the development of MODS. All found tissue changes were unspecific;
they were caused by disorders in the blood circulation system, cytotoxic

---

* Email: lebedinska@mail.ru.

and fibroplastic effects. These changes created preconditions for the development of multi-organ failure in animals, after they were injected with endotoxin of E. coli. It should be noted that observed pathologic changes in organs caused by LPS are similar to diagnosed changes in the samples tissues of the patients with multi-organ failure, caused by SIRS. This fact shows a significant role of bacterial endotoxins in multi-organ failure development.

PATHOMORPHOLOGICAL PECULIARITIES OF SEPSIS IN CANCER PATIENTS

Morphological study has determined meaning for postmortal confirmation of clinically diagnosed sepsis and that's why it requires a detailed description of damaged organs and confirmation of the presence of infection. Also it should be noted that often there is no correspondence between histological data and the degree of organ dysfunction in patients who died because of sepsis. Death of cells in heart, kidneys, liver and lungs can be slight and it will not show the degree of organ dysfunction. Usually there are local lesions with normal structure of uriniferous tubules and renal glomerulus in patients with sepsis and acute renal insufficiency [1]. It accords to the alterations in patients with isolated renal insufficiency, where we observe a discrepancy between the degree of necrosis of uriniferous tubules and a degree of dysfunction [2]. It seems that there are no massive deaths of renal cells during the sepsis, because functions of kidneys normalize in most patients that survived sepsis and renal insufficiency [1]. Obviously most organ dysfunctions can be explained by «cell hibernation» or «cell stunning» as it happens during myocardial ischemia [3]. It seems that sepsis activates protection mechanisms that reduce cellular processes to housekeeping functions. Fink et al. 2002 wrote that the reducing of oxygen consumption caused by endogenous oxidant is the basis of molecular explanation of cellular stunning [4,5]. It is considered that organ (multi organ) failure is connected with proven or supposed bacteremia («septicemia») [6], but there is no confirmed standard of hystopathologic characteristics that indicate septicemia. That's why combinations of clinical, laboratorial and morphological study are used to confirm sepsis. It should be noted that morphological signs of septicemia are seldom noticed and interpretation of premortal and especially postmortal analysis of blood is very difficult. That is the reason why data from an autopsy does not coincide with a clinical diagnosis in spite of modern methods of study. The last studies showed that discrepancies between diagnoses based on clinical symptoms and morphological changes were in 16-32% of cases, mostly in immune-compromised patients and in patients with fungal infections. After the autopsy of patients with undiagnosed diseases – malignant tumors, myocardial infarction, endocarditis, and pulmonary embolisms were found. In studies about sepsis it is noted that vital diagnosis of sepsis can be insufficient or excessive [7, 8]. Though a morphological study for diagnosis of sepsis is very important, autopsies were performed in only 7.7% cases of deaths recorded in the reanimations resuscitation department in European clinics. The autopsies showed that main entrances for sepsis are pneumonia and different infections – intravascular (including endocarditis and catheter-associated infections), abdominal, surgical, and urological. However, the detection of histological signs of sepsis do not always mean that the patient died from sepsis.

Microbiological Studies

The role of detection of bacteremia in the diagnostics of sepsis is ambiguous, because it is not always clear if the reason is sepsis or transient pervasion of microorganisms into blood flow. So it is important to understand if the sequences of syndromes of sepsis depend on the initial infection. One of the problems in autopsying patients with sepsis is the absence of confirming procedures for taking, conserving, and transporting biological samples with minimal contamination from the external environment. There also may be postmortal penetration of bacteria from the intestines into blood. Interpretation of positive results of bacteriologic studies is often complicated by the second contamination of the biological samples by microorganisms. At the same time identification of such bacteria as Mycobacterium, Streptococcus groups A (pyogenes), Streptococcus pneumonia and Neisseria meningitis is not likely to be accidental or a consequence of contamination.

Sepsis-like Illness

When performing an autopsy on patients with clinical signs of sepsis or undetected infection it is necessary to compare the differential diagnostics with the following clinically similar illnesses: disseminated tumors (for example, lung micro-embolism as a result of cancer can cause obstruction of lung arterioles and cause cardiorespiratory insufficiency); thrombotic microangiopathy; multi-organ atherosclerosis; burns; adrenal insufficiency; pancreatitis; thyroid storm; trauma; coronary artery bypass; heat stroke; hypersensitivity reaction and anaphylaxis.

Pathomorphological Characteristics of Organs in Patients with Sepsis

Heart

Dysfunctions of the myocardium connected with sepsis are the decrease of cardiac output and increasing heart rate [9]. Morphological changes are apoptotic changes in cardiomyocytes, hyperemia, and blood stasis (Figure 2.1).

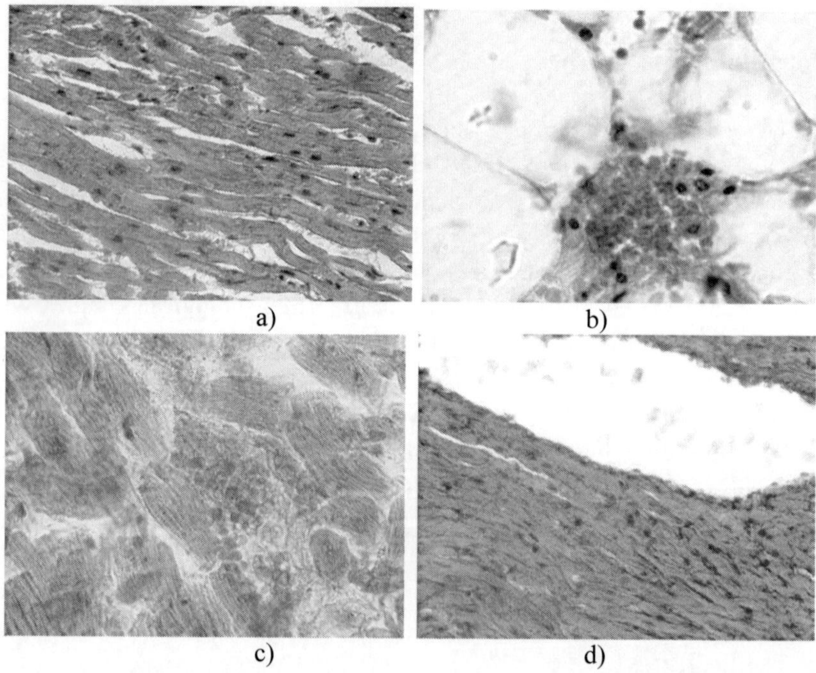

Figure 2.1. Pathomorphological changes in myocardium of patients with sepsis. Haemotoxylin-eosin staining. a) Apoptotic changes in cardiomyocytes. Original magnification 400; b) Blood stasis in vessels. Cluster of macrophages around the vessel. Original magnification 900; c) Damage of cadiomyocytes. Interstitial macrophages between cardiomyocytes. Original magnification 900; d) Generalized activation of endothelial cells during sepsis. Original magnification 400.

Pathomorphologic study of the heart also detects infiltration of lymphocytes and histiocytes in myocardium. Leucocytic infiltration is considered to be the consequence of capillary permeability as a result of generalized activation of endothelial cells with appearance of inter-endothelial nexus (toxic cardiomyopathy). However, we usually don't observe defects of the myocardium in patients that survived sepsis. It seems that heart dysfunction is caused by an excessive amount of cytokines and myocardium hypoperfusion and it can be reversed. [10]. Taking into consideration weakly expressed changes in the myocardium, the recommendation is to study at least 5 samples of heart tissues: 2 from the right and 3 from the left ventriculums [11].

Brain

Light microscopy does not allow detection of changes in the brains of patients with sepsis or septic shock. In spite of the small amount of research in this area we can confirm that transient changes in the brains of patients are caused by inflammation mediators [9]. Expressed pathologic changes in the brain are secondary and they are connected with sepsis complications including: cerebral infarction caused by thromboembolic, hypoxic/ischemic encephalopathy after temporary stop of blood flow or/and oxygen supply; metastatic brain abscess or/and meningitis from remote sepsis focus; cerebral micro infarction. The most sensitive zones of the brain to ischemic damage are the cerebellar nuclei, hippocampus and cortex [12].

Lung

Dysfunction of the lung at the first stage of severe sepsis can be observed in approximately 20% of patients [9]. Acute pulmonary insufficiency is diagnosed if there is arterial hypoxemia ($PaO_2/FiO_2 < 300$mm Hg) and if an X-ray study discovers double-sided pulmonary infiltration without pneumonia or cardiac arrest. This condition is defined as acute respiratory distress syndrome (ARDS) or diffuse alveolar damage (DAD). These syndromes are not specific for sepsis because the same changes can be observed after inhalation poisoning (poison gas, smoke, high concentration of oxygen et al.), after aspiration of stomach contents or after radiation-induced damage. DAD also can be an indicator of SIRS caused by ejection of mediators into blood flow without development of an infectious process, caused by the presence of inflammation mediators. DAD can also be caused by cytostatic treatment, pancreatitis, cardio-pulmonary anastomosis, system shock of any origin, blood transfusion reactions, fat embolism, intoxication by herbicides, and other reasons [13].

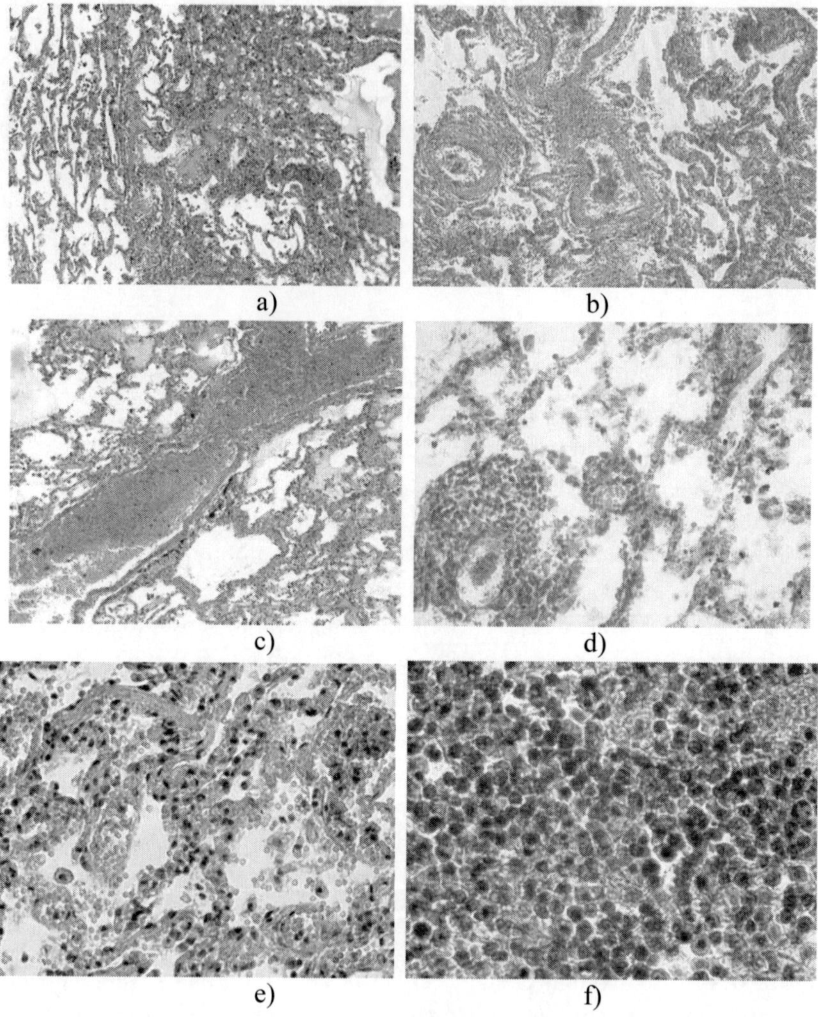

Figure 2.2. Pathomorphological changes in lung of patients with sepsis at exudative stage. Haemotoxylin-eosin staining. a, b) Blood stasis, thickening of alveolar walls, effusion of blood and edema in lung tissue. Original magnification 100; c) Blood stasis in vessels, thickening of alveolar walls, blood effusion and edema in lung tissue. Original magnification 200; d) Perivascular leucocytic infiltration. Original magnification 200; e) Leucocytic infiltration of alveolar walls. Original magnification 400; f) Area of neutrophilic infiltration of lung tissue. Original magnification 400.

DAD has stages called exudative, regenerative and reparational. The exudative stage lasts approximately 1 week: lungs become dark red and heavier. This stage is characterized by widening of alveolar walls, hyperemia, edema, presence of neutrophils in the interstitium and erythrocytes in the alveolus (Figure 2.2). Damage of the alveolar epithelium is usually not observed by light microscopy. After the exudative stage there is a stage called "shock lung". It appears as alveolar collapse, blood effusions and edema, formation of hyaline membranes (fibrin and necrotic epithelial cells) on the epithelial surface of respiratory bronchiole and acinus, stasis of neutrophils in capillaries of alveolar walls (Figure 2.3).

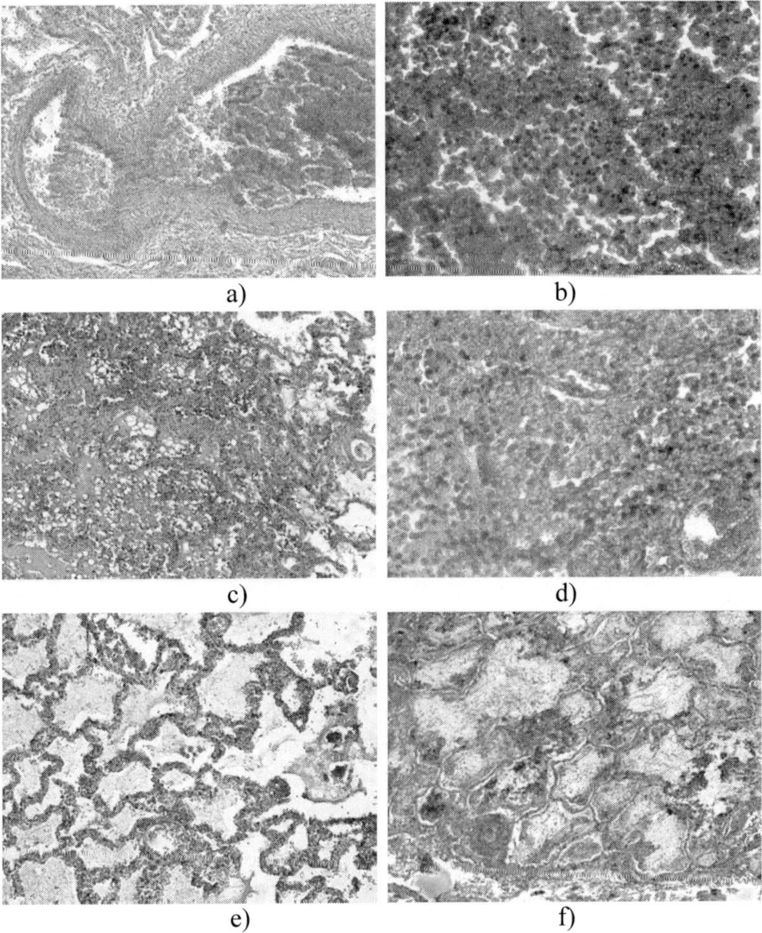

a)   b)

c)   d)

e)   f)

Figure 2.3. (Continued).

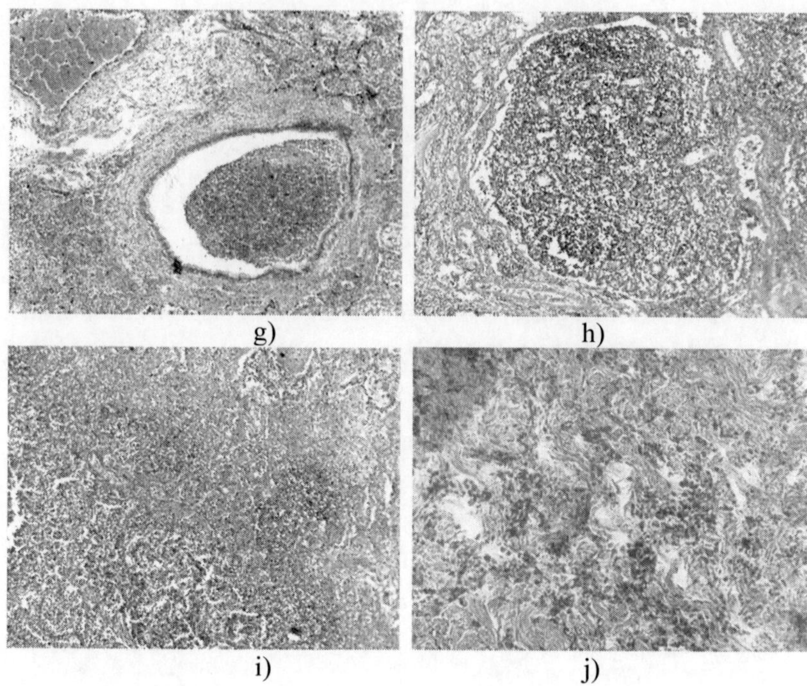

Figure 2.3. Pathomorphological changes in lungs of patients with sepsis at the stage called "shock lung". Haemotoxylin-eosin staining. a) Blood stasis in large vessels. Original magnification 100 b) Blood stasis in capillaries, blood effusion into lung tissues. Original magnification 100 c) Alveolar collapse, blood effusion and edema of lung. Original magnification 100 d) Blood stasis in vessels, blood effusions into lung tissues during sepsis. Original magnification 200 e, f). Formation of hyaline membranes on the epithelial surface of respiratory bronchioles and acinus. Original magnification 200 and 400 respectively. g, h, i) Blood stasis in the vessels, leucocytic embolism in vessels, stasis of neutrophils in the capillaries of alveolar walls. Original magnification 100 j) Stasis of neutrophils in the capillaries of alveolar walls. Original magnification 400.

During the regenerative stage the restoration of the native structure of the lung or development of the process with formation of fibrosis may occur. Epithelial cells proliferate actively and replace damaged epithelium. They become large and elongate like lung macrophages. The epithelium can grow under/on the hyaline membrane, growing into the alveolar wall and forming interstitial fibrosis. In the capillaries the damage of the endothelium sometimes causes local thrombosis, formation of new vessels and local vessel reconstruction. The reparative stage starts only if there was no tissue damage over the time phase of regeneration. Progressive thinning of interstitial tissue of alveolar walls is observed. Incorporation of hyaline membranes and pervasion of fibroblasts cause organization of effusion. Granulation tissue is formed in the alveoli, as in pneumonia in the stage of organization. Fibrosis can occur in a few weeks.

Neutropenic Sepsis

In most cases this terminal condition is observed in cancer patients after antineoplastic therapy. There are bacteria in many organs and blood vessels of these patients; alveoli in lungs are filled with fibrin and mononuclear leucocytes (Figure 2.4).

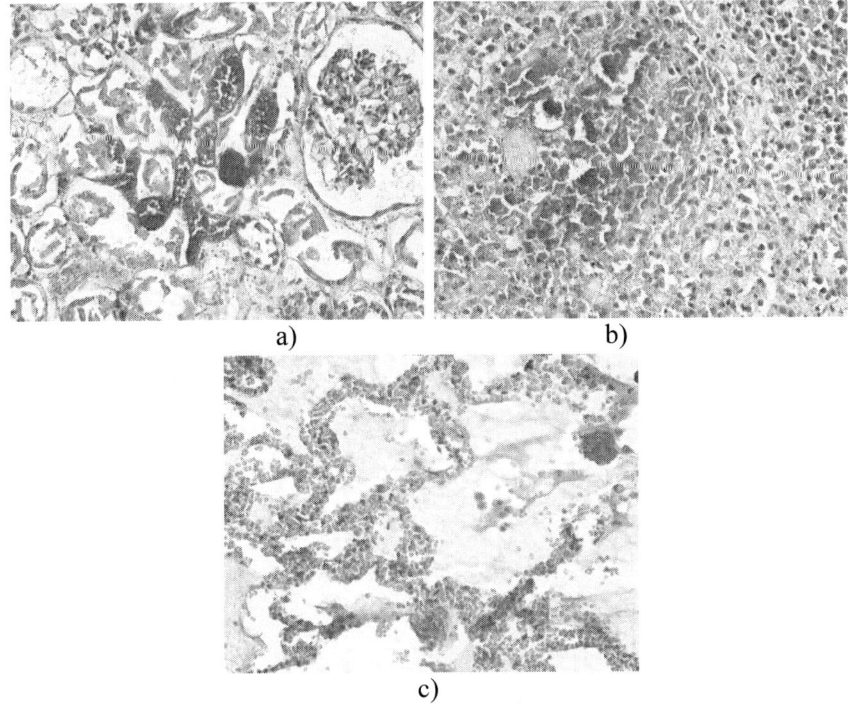

Figure 2.4. Changes in the micromorphology of kidney, lung and liver of the patient with neutropenic sepsis. Haemotoxylin-eosin staining. Original magnification 400; a) Kidney. Bacterial embolia, dystrophy of renal epithelium of tubuli. b) Liver. Bacterial embolia, dystrophy of hepatocytes, disorganization of lobules, blood stasis in the vessels. c) Lung. Bacterial embolia, fibrin and mononuclear leucocytes in alveoli.

Liver

In the patients with sepsis and septic shock, the liver usually does not have specific morphological features. But if the source of sepsis is the bile duct inflammation abscesses can be found clustered in the portal tract area of the liver. In that case the liver is heavier than normal, has softer consistency, and there is cholestasis. The microstructure is characterized by autolysis of hepatocytes with disintegration of liver bars and lobuli (Figure 2.5). Also steatosis and small leucocytic infiltrates are often observed. The hemophagocytosis can be seen.

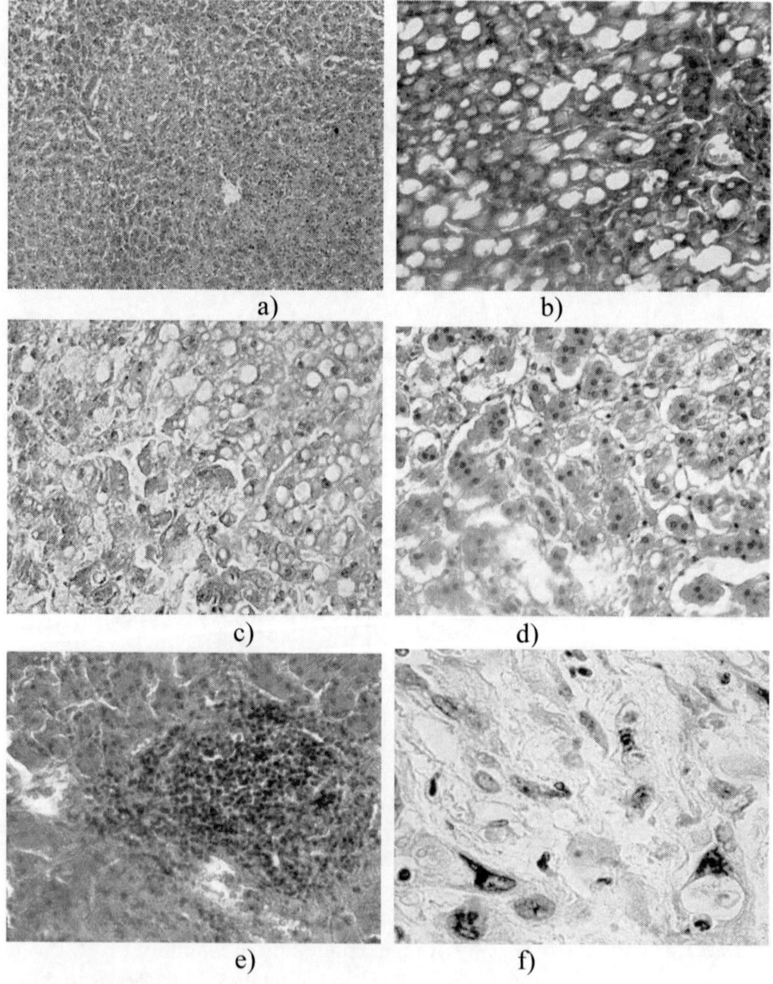

Figure 2.5. (Continued).

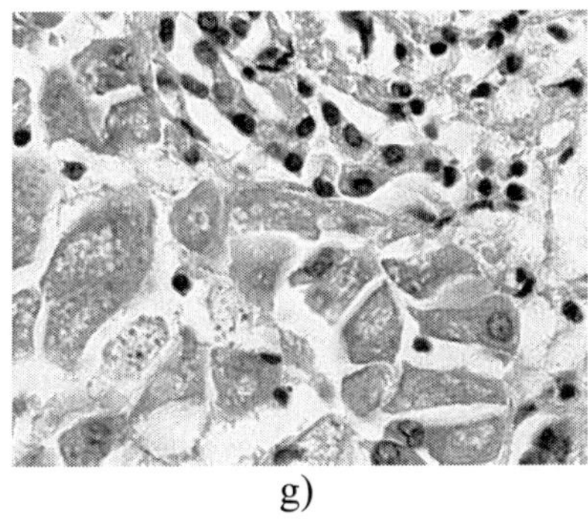

g)

Figure 2.5. Pathomorphological changes in liver of patients with sepsis. a) Blood stasis in sinusoidal capillaries, disintegration of liver bars and lobules. Haemotoxylin-eosin staining. Original magnification 100; b) Fatty degeneration of hepatocytes. Disintegration of liver bars and lobuli. Haemotoxylin-eosin staining. Original magnification 400; c) Fatty degeneration and autolysis of hepatocytes. Disintegration of liver bars. Van-Gieson staining. Original magnification 400; d) Apoptosis of hepatocytes. Disintegration of liver bars. Haemotoxylin-eosin staining. Original magnification 400; e) Intra lobular leucocytic infiltration. Disintegration of bars and lobules. Haemotoxylin-eosin staining. Original magnification 400; f) Destruction of hepatocytes. Activation of endotheliocytes and Kupffer cells. Methylene blue staining. Original magnification 900; g) Autolysis of hepatocytes. Activation of endotheliocytes and Kupffer cells. Haemotoxylin-eosin staining. Original magnification 900.

Kidney

Acute renal failure (ARF) is observed in 20% of patients with sepsis and in 50% of patients with septic shock [9]. ARF in the most frequent organ failure that is indicated by oliguria and azotaemia. Pathogenesis of the illness is indicated by system hypotonia, vasoconstriction of the vessels in the kidney. In this state the organ is susceptible to the toxic influence of the drugs or endogenous inflammation mediators and pathologic changes characterize the acute damage of tubuli (ADT or acute tubular necrosis). Kidneys are significantly enlarged (edema of cortical layer) and are pale with unclear cortical-medullar borders, local abscesses, ascending acute pyelonephritis and infarction of the cortical layer. Renal glomeruli can be collapsed but also can be without signs of damage. Damage of tubuli can be toxic and of ischemic origin [15]. In septic shock the differences between them become unclear. The main characteristics of ADT are interstitial edema with tubuli separation and swelling of the tubular epithelium, loss of the nucleus of epithelial cells, apoptosis, desquamation of tubular epithelium, thinning of the epithelium, regeneration of tubular cells (appearance of hyperchromic enlarged nucleus and mitosis), interstitial inflammation, accumulation of lymphocytes, myeloid precursors, precursors of erythrocytes between the tubuli (Figure 2.6).

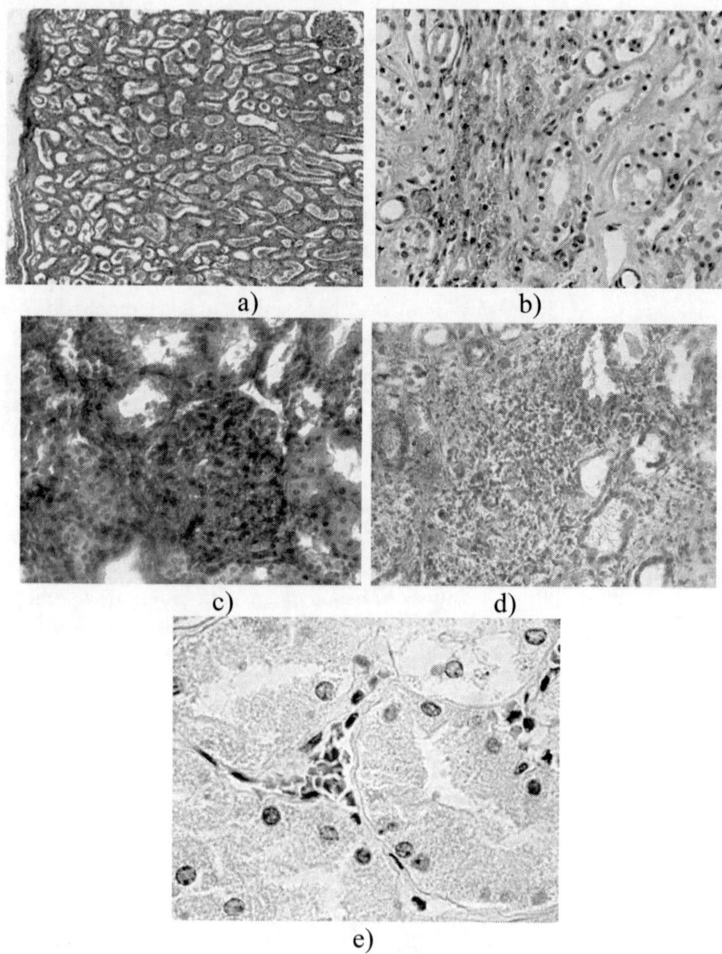

Figure 2.6. Pathomorphological changes in kidneys of patients with sepsis. a) Blood stasis in the vessels, desquamation of tubular epithelium in the patient with sepsis. Van-Gieson staining. Original magnification 100 b) Blood stasis in the vessels, desquamation of tubular epithelium. Van-Gieson staining. Original magnification 200 c) Blood stasis in the vessels of the renal glomerulus, desquamation of epithelium. Haemotoxylin-Eosin staining. Original magnification 400 d) Interstitial edema and inflammation. Blood stasis in the vessels, desquamation of tubular epithelium. Haemotoxylin-Eosin staining. Original magnification 200 e) Desquamation of tubular epitheliumin. Haemotoxylin-Eosin staining. Original magnification 900.

Microvesicular vacuolization of proximal tubuli is not a sign of the acute tubular injury. It can be the result of applying drugs containing dextrose. Late autopsy does not reveal these features. After the death of the patient the kidneys must be examined as soon as possible, because they are susceptible to autolysis.

Adrenal Glands

Adrenal glands of people who died because of sepsis may have the following features: depletion of lipids or hyperplasia, atrophy caused by prolonged treatment by steroid drugs, blood effusion (small or drain), thrombosis in arterioles (Figure 2.7).

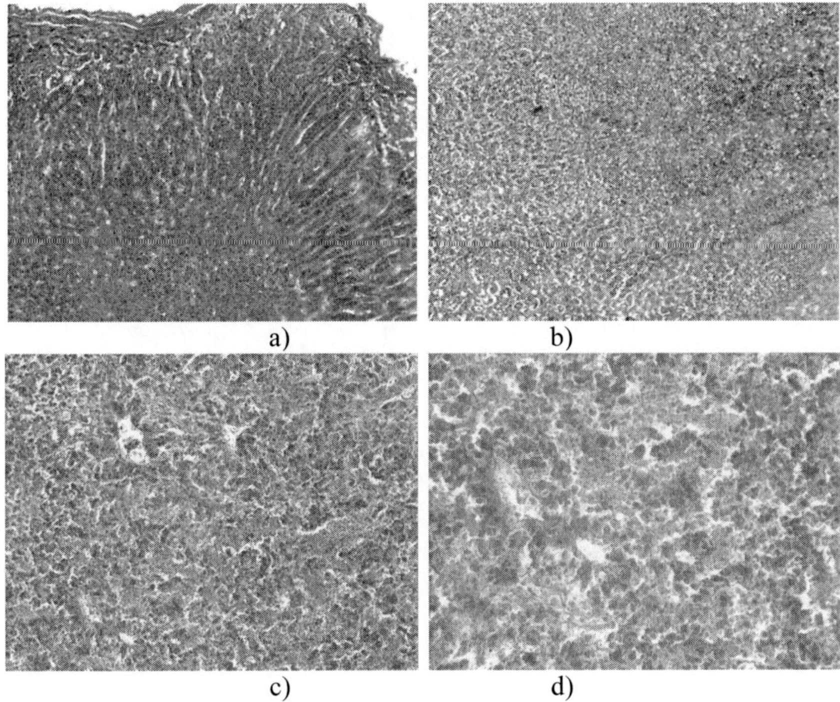

Figure 2.7. Pathomorphological changes in adrenal glands of patients with sepsis. Haemotoxylin-eosin staining. a, b) Hyperplasia, blood effusion and thrombosis of the vessels in the patient with sepsis . Original magnification 100 c, d) Hyperplasia, blood effusion and thrombosis of vessels in the patient with sepsis. Original magnification 200 and 400 respectively.

Hemophagocytic Syndrome

Hemophagocytic syndrome (HS) is the illness where there is an excessive phagocytosis of blood elements in the bone marrow, spleen and lymph nodes by macrophages (Figure 2.8). It is caused by hyper activation of macrophages during the pathologic processes like sepsis or SIRS. Distinctive feature of HS is non-regulated phagocytosis of blood cells and their precursors. This syndrome is accompanied by fever, pancytopenia, liver failure, hepatosplenomegaly, hyperferritinemia, blood clotting disorder including fibrin degradation and fibrinopenia.

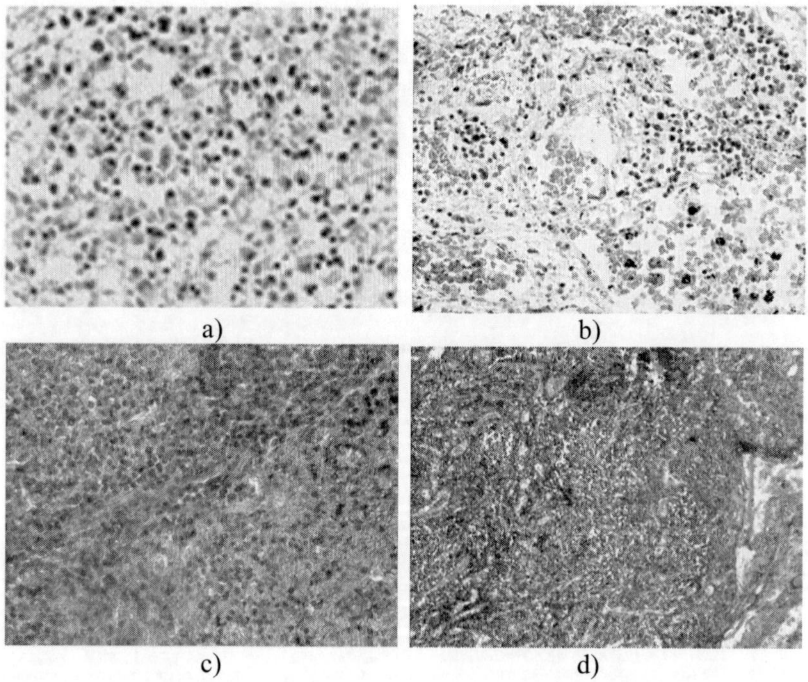

Figure 2.8. Hemophagocytosis in the tissues of the internal organs of a patient with sepsis. Haemotoxylin-Eosin staining. a) Bone marrow. Hemophagocytosis in the patient with sepsis. Many macrophages have captured red blood cells. Original magnification 200 b, c) Spleen. Hemophagocytosis in the patient with sepsis. Many macrophages have captured hemosiderin. Original magnification 200 d) Lymph node. Many hemosiderophages. Original magnification 100.

A combination of HS with septic shock is associated with 70% lethality [15]. Many patients have HS and SIRS without detecting the infection. HS pathogenesis is considered as an aberrant excessive immune reaction with overactivation of macrophages by cytokines (especially TNF, IL-6,IL-1, IFNγ) and as a result of T-cells activation. Hemophagocytosis in T-cells is discovered in one third of patients who died in the reanimation. It is frequently revealed in patients with sepsis and after blood transfusion, but it is not discovered in patients with cardiovascular diseases.

Thrombotic Microangiopathy

Thrombus consists of fibrin and platelets in different proportions. During the time of sepsis and other diseases thrombi frequently are clustered in small vessels. During disseminated intravascular coagulation, thrombi consist mainly of fibrin. This process is accompanied by coagulopathy and depletion of coagulation factors in blood [16]. The renal glomerulus and alveolar capillaries in lungs are the most frequent places for the microthrombus position (Figure 2.9).

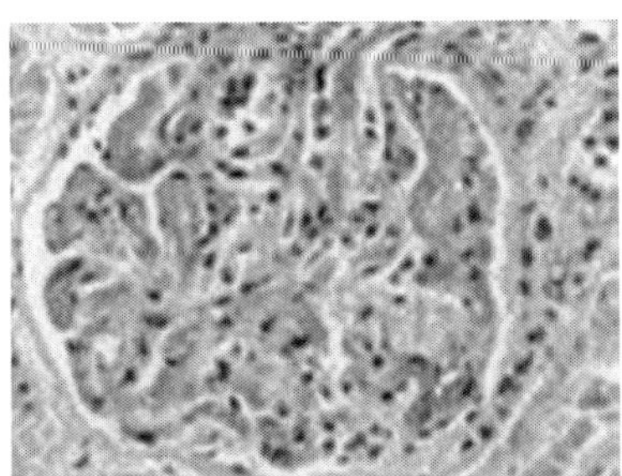

Figure 2.9. Kidney. Fibrin thrombi in the capillaries of renal glomerulus in the patient with meningococcus sepsis.

Apoptosis of Immunocompetent Cells and Epithelial Cells in the Patients with Sepsis

In most patients with sepsis apoptosis, it is mainly discovered in 2 types of cells: lymphocytes and epithelial cells of the digestive tract. This data coincides with the data acquired from the experiments on animals [1]. Normally lymphocytes and epitheliocytes in the digestive tract are renewed quickly. The main mechanism of cellular death is apoptosis. Sepsis seems to accelerate these physiological processes. Focal necroses of hepatocytes around central veins (the most susceptible to hypoxia) are often found in the brains and hearts of patients with sepsis.

Generally the performed study of patients established the presence of multi-organ failure (MOF), caused by non-specific changes of microstructure of organs, which obviously caused the death of patients. The most significant changes can be observed in the tissue of the lungs, kidneys and liver after the histological study of tissue samples taken from cancer patients who died because of sepsis. Disseminated intravascular coagulation was observed in all organs. Erythrocytic, fibrinous, and leucocytic thrombi were observed in blood vessels in different organs. Signs of intravascular coagulation caused the appearance of many foci of necrosis in tissues because of thrombosis and blood effusions with different sizes. Atrophy of lymphatic tissue and degenerative changes of cardimyocytes and endotheliocytes of myocardial vessels.

STUDY OF THE PATHOGENETIC ROLE OF E. COLI LPS IN THE DEVELOPMENT OF MULTI-ORGAN FAILURE IN EXPERIMENTS ON LABORATORY ANIMALS

A series of special experiments performed in collaboration with Dr. N. Yu. Anisimova was performed to prove the pathogenetic influence of microorganism toxins, especially LPS in the development of MODS. Solution of E. coli LPS was injected into the mice intraperitoneally. After 48 hours we observed significant damage of microstructure in all studied organs (kidneys, liver, heart, spleen, lungs). The most significant changes were observed in lungs, liver and kidneys. All changes were unspecific and were caused by disorders in blood microcirculation. They obviously created preconditions for the development of organ and multi-organ failures after the injection of endotoxin. It should be noted that observed pathologic changes of organs during toxicosis induced by LPS, which are not accompanied by bacteremia or fungemia, are similar to changes of tissue of internal organs of patients with sepsis and MODS [18]. This fact shows the significant, and perhaps main role of bacterial endotoxins in the development of this syndrome and confirms the theory about the opportunity of development of the clinical signs similar to sepsis (sepsis – like syndrome) with the absence of primary and secondary bacterial infection, weakening of barrier functions of the mucosa and skin.

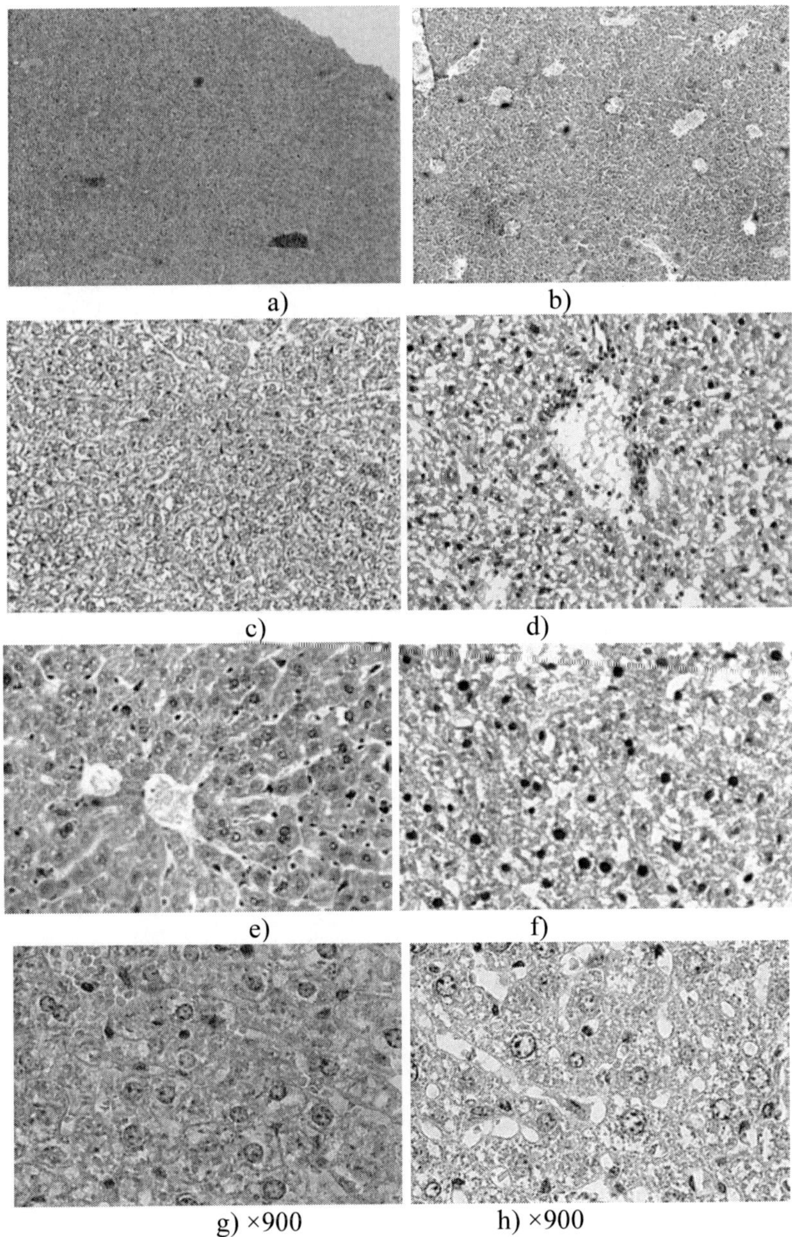

Figure 2.10. Morphologic changes in mouse liver after injection of LPS E. coli (right column) compared with intact control (left column). Haemotoxilin-eosin staining. a, b - original magnification 100; c, d-original magnification 200; e,f - original magnification 400;g,h - original magnification 900.

It is known that endotoxemia, especially that detected by the presence of LPS in blood flow, can develop by stress genic transintestinal translocation, which can be caused by surgery in particular [19-21]. We should probably agree with the opinion of prof. V.K. Kozlov (2006) that sepsis can't be considered an unconnected nosological unit (disease); it should be considered as a variant of a complicated clinical condition of infectious and non-infectious origin, which causes SIRS [22]. If there are signs of SIRS then high susceptibility to sepsis is obvious.

A solution of E. coli LPS (Sigma) was injected into CBA line mice intraperitoneally, 2 times with 24-hour intervals, 3 mg/mouse. 24 hours after the second injection of bacterial endotoxin the mice were euthanized and their kidneys, lungs, spleens and hearts were taken for histological study. 48 hours later, after the injection of E. coli endotoxin, significant damage of the microstructure was observed in all studied organs. Pathological changes were the most significant in lungs, liver and kidneys.

Morphologic changes in the liver (Figure 2.10) were probably caused by activation of Kupffer cells and increased the size of the endotheliocytes and their nuclei in sinusoidal capillaries. Platelets created clusters inside the vessels. In the hepatocytes many signs of degeneration and focal necroses were observed. Perivascular edema, necroses of hepatocytes around the areas of necrosis-cellular infiltrates of granular leucocytes, lymphocytes and macrophages were found. Sludge, microthrombi, fatty degeneration of hepatocytes, and central vein walls infiltrated with leucocytes were also detected.

Pathomorphological study of lungs showed significant decrease of lung tissue aeriness (Figure 2.11). We also noticed interstitial edema of lung tissue with neutrophilic infiltration of the lung wall, hyperemia and atelectasis, foci of alveolar blood effusions and necrosis with significant amounts of hemosiderin, and activation of lung macrophages. There was a lot of sludge in the bronchi and bronchioli, and desquamation of mucosa epithelium. In addition, we noted lymphocytic infiltration, vessel disorders, fibroblast proliferation, foci of necrosis and emphysema.

Also, significant hemodynamical and metabolical changes were found in kidneys of mice from the experimental group. From Figure 2.12 we can see degenerative changes and necrosis of epithelial cells in proximal and distal tubuli. Hyperemia of capillaries in renal glomeruli was also observed. There was desquamation of the epithelium and sludge in the tubuli.

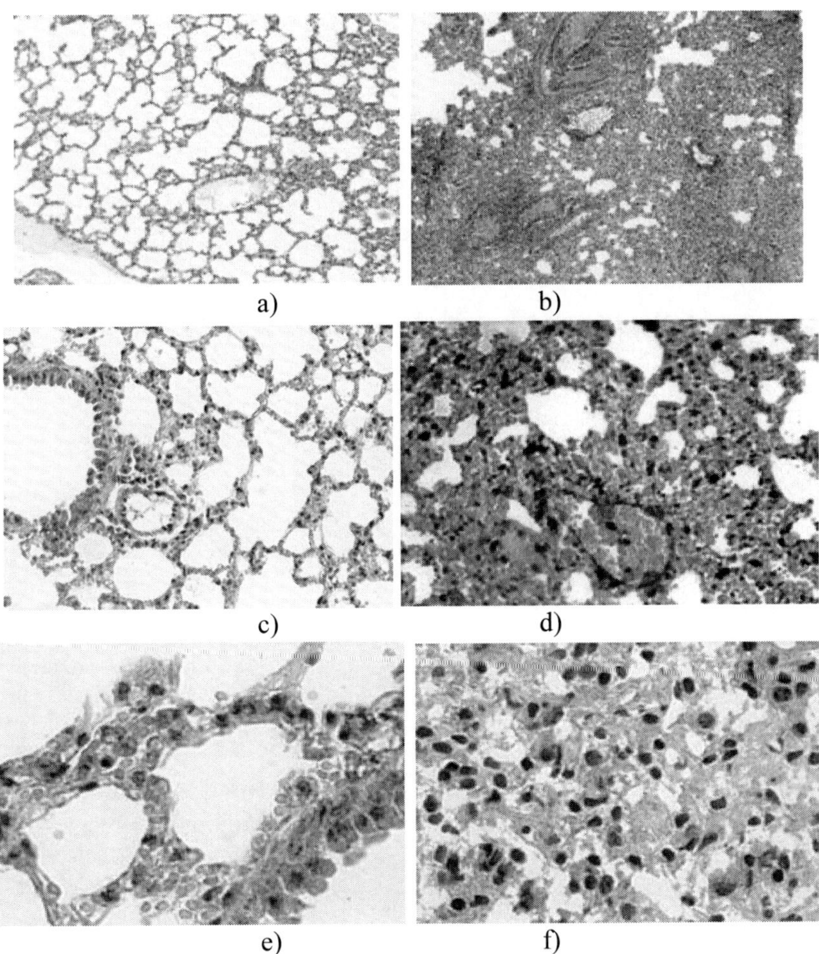

Figure 2.11. Morphologic changes in lung of mouse after injection of E. coli LPS (right column) compared with intact control (left column). Haemotoxilin-eosin staining.
a, b - original magnification 200; c, d-original magnification 400; e,f-original magnification 900.

Compared with other studied organs, the spleen had less significant morphological changes after injection of LPS. Experimental group animals had blood stasis in the organ's vessels (Figure 2.13) Also there was a slight depletion of lymphoid cells in white pulp and a decrease of lymphoid node size.

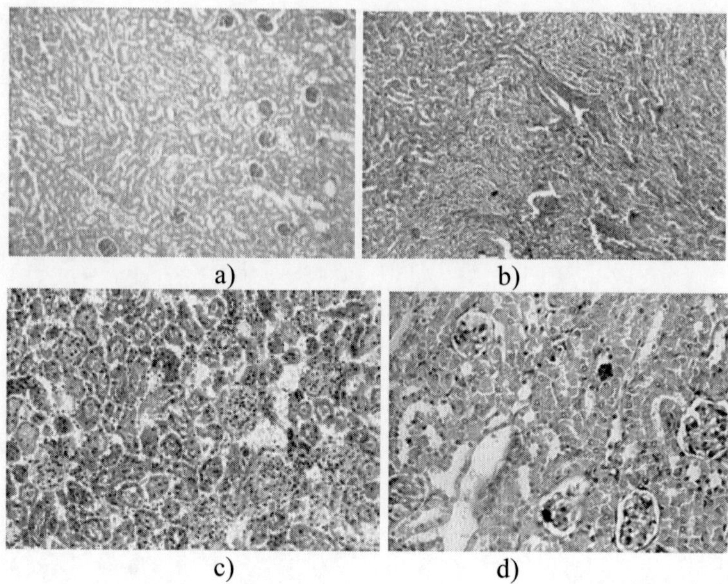

Figure 2.12. Morphologic changes in mouse kidneys after E. coli LPS injection (right column) compared with intact control (left column). Haemotoxylin-eosin staining. a, b - original magnification 100; c, d-original magnification 200; e,f - original magnification 400.

All found changes were unspecific, they were caused by disorders in the blood circulation system and had cytotoxic and fibroplastic effects. These changes created preconditions for the development of multi-organ failure in animals after they were injected with endotoxin of E. coli. It should be noted that observed pathologic changes in organs caused by LPS are similar to diagnosed changes in the sample tissues of patients with multi-organ failure, caused by SIRS.

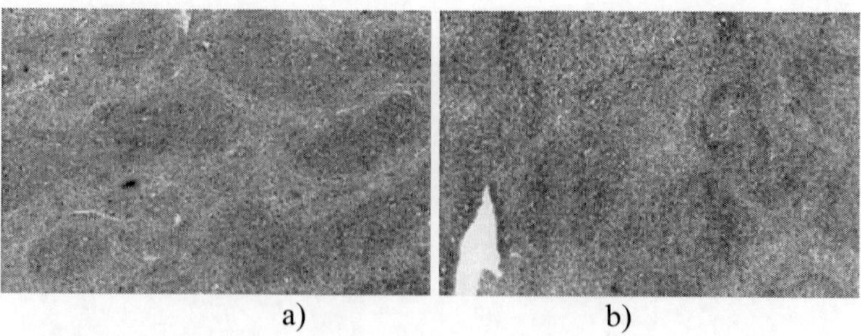

Figure 2.13. (Continued).

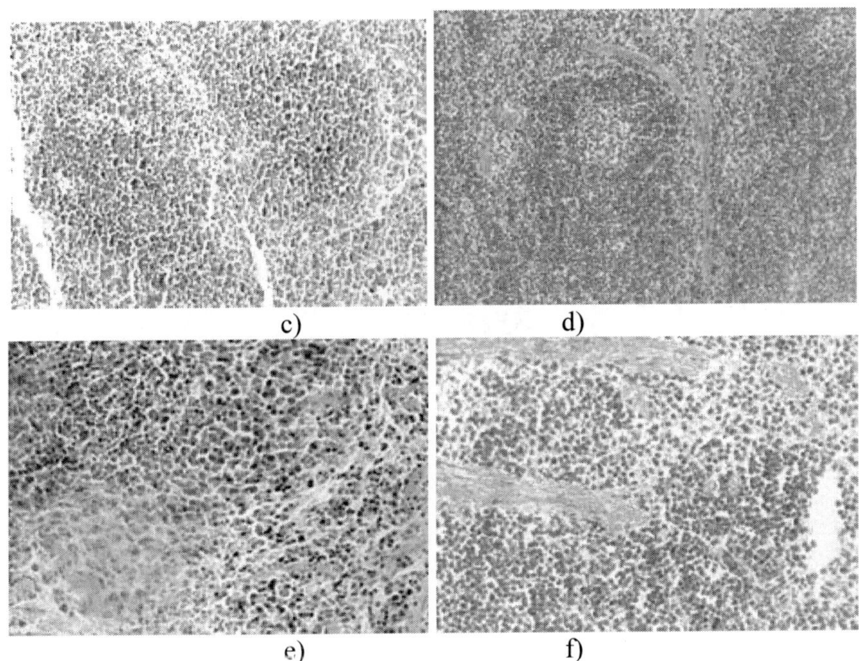

Figure 2.13. Morphologic changes in mouse spleen after E. coli LPS injection (right column) compared with intact control (left column). Haemotoxylin-eosin staining. a, b - original magnification 100; c, d-original magnification 200; e,f - original magnification 400.

This fact shows a significant role of bacterial endotoxins in multi-organ failure development and confirms the theory about the opportunistic appearance of clinical signs similar to sepsis (sepsis-like syndrome) without the presence of bacterial infection during the weakening of barrier functions of mucosa and skin. Endotoxemia, indicated by the presence of E. coli LPS in the blood flow can develop because of stressogenic transintestinal translocation.

CONCLUSION

We can suppose that well-timed effective elimination of bacterial endotoxins from the blood flow can significantly decrease development of system pathological changes in organ tissue, caused by disorders in microcirculation. This will prevent the development of multi-organ failure. Acquired data allow us to suppose that triggers (microorganisms and their toxins) and mediators of inflammation, secreted by immuno-competent cells, play an important role in pathogenesis of sepsis and SIRS. It seems to be reasonable to recommend additional extracorporeal methods of detofixication in the standard treatment for patients for elimination of bacteria and their toxins from the blood flow and decreasing the cascade of inflammation mediators.

REFERENCES

[1]   Hotchkiss, R; Swanson, P; Freeman, B. Apoptotic cell death in patients with sepsis, shock, and multiple organ dysfunction. *Crit. Care Med.*1999 V.27, pp 1230–1251.

[2]   Weinberg, J; Venkatachalam, M. Guanine nucleotides and acute renal failure. *J. Clin. Invest.* 2001 V.108,pp 1279–1281.

[3]   Sawyer, D; Loscalzo, J. Myocardial hibernation: restorative or preterminal sleep? *Circulation.* 2002 V.105, pp 1517–1519.

[4]   Khan, A; Delude,R;Han, Y.et al. Liposomal NAD(+) prevents diminished O(2) consumption by immuno-stimulated Caco-2 cells. *Am. J. Physiol. Lung Cell Mol. Physiol.* 2002 V.282, pp 1082–1091.

[5]   Fink, MP. Bench-to-bedside review: Cytopathic hypoxia. *Crit Care.* 2002 V.6 (6), pp 491-499.

[6]   Lucas, S. The autopsy pathology of sepsis-related death. *Current Diagnostic Pathology.* 2007 V. 13, pp 375–388.

[7]   Perkins, G; McAuley, D; Davies, S; Gao, F. Discrepancies between clinical and postmortem diagnoses in critically ill patients: an observational study. *Crit Care.* 2003 V.7(6), pp 129–132.

[8]   Blosser, S; Zimmerman, H; Stauffer, J. Do autopsies of critically ill patients reveal important findings that were clinically undetected? *Crit Care Med.*-1998 V.26(8), pp 1332–1336.

[9]   Munford, R; Pugin, J. Normal responses to injury prevent systemic inflammation and can be immunosuppressive. *Am. J. Respir. Crit. Care Med.* 2001 V.163, pp 316–321.

[10] Levi M. Current understanding of disseminated intravascular coagulation. *Br. J. Haematol.* 2004 V. 124(5), pp 567–576.

[11] Royal College of Pathologists. Sudden death with likely cardiac pathology. Guidelines for Autopsy Practice-best practice scenarios, 2005.

[12] Whitwell, H(2005).Techniques. In: H. Whitwell, Editor, *Forensic neuropathology*, Hodder Arnold, London pp. 20–35.

[13] Corrin, B. Diffuse alveolar damage. In: Evans TW, Haslett C, ed. ARDS Acute Respiratory Distress in Adults, London: Chapman & Hall Medical. 1996 pp37-46.

[14] Racusen, L, Kashgarian, M (2007). Ischemic and toxic acute tubular injury and other ischemic renal injury. In: *Pathology of the Kidney*, 6th ed., edited by Jennette JC, Olson JL, Schwartz MM, Silva FG, Philadelphia, Lippincott Williams & Wilkins, pp 1139 –1198.

[15] Fisman, D. Hemophagocytic syndromes and infection. *Emerg. Infect. Dis*. 2000 V.6 (6), pp 601–608.

[16] Toh, C. Characterization of thrombin activatable fibrinolysis inhibitor in normal and acquired haemostatic dysfunction. *Blood.Coagul. Fibrinolysis*. 2003 V.14(1), pp 69–71.

[17] Bateman, R; Sharpe M; Ellis C. Bench-to-bedside review: microvascular dysfunction in sepsis—hemodynamics, oxygen transport, and nitric oxide. *Crit. Care Med*. 2003 V.7,pp 359–373.

[18] Anisimova, NYu. Pathogenetic reasons for use of extracorporeal detoxification of cancer patients with sepsis. *Dr. Sci. Thesis*, Moscow; 2012.

[19] Isakov, Yu F, Beloborodova NV. Sepsis in children. Mokeev 2001.

[20] Balzan, S; Quadros, CDA; Cleva, RD; Zilberstein, B; Cecconello, I. Bacterial translocation: Overview of mechanisms and clinical impact. *Issue J. Gastroenterol. Hepatol*. 2007, V. 22(4), pp 464–471.

[21] Deitch, E.A; Bridges R.M. Effect of stress and trauma on bacterial translocation from the gut. *J. SurgRes* 1987 V. 42 (5), pp 536–542.

[22] Kozlov, VK. Sepsis, etiology, immunopathogenesis, conception of modern immunetherapy. S- Petersburg. Dialekt 2006.

Chapter 3

USE OF HEMOSORPTION IN TREATMENT OF CANCER PATIENTS: EFFECTIVENESS OF DIFFERENT DEVICES

N. Yu. Anisimova[*], A. Yu. Grebenko, E. G. Gromova,
L. S. Kuznetsova and M. V. Kiselevsky

N.N. Blokhin Russian Cancer Research Center, Russian Academy of
Medical Sciences, Kashirskoe Sh, 24, 115478, Moscow,
Russian Federation

ABSTRACT

Understanding the significant role of the triggers and mediators of SIRS cascade in development of MODS, it seems to be reasonable to include extracorporeal detoxification methods of treatment in complex therapy of cancer patients with sepsis. These methods provide effective elimination of bacterial toxins and excess of circulating microbial molecules from the systemic blood flow, which play a crucial role in the development of systemic inflammatory response. This chapter will summarize the results of our studies on the effectiveness of different extracorporeal methods (hemosorption, hemodialysis, hemodiafiltration, hemofiltration) in the treatment of cancer patients with sepsis. It was shown, that non-selective hemosorption and selective hemosorption provided more efficient elimination of bacterial lipopolysaccharide and

---

[*] Corresponding author: Email: n.u.anisimova@gmail.com.

mediators of inflammation from peripheral blood than previously used methods of filtration. That is accompanied by normalization of the functional activity of innate immunity effectors and decreased the severity of the patients' condition and increased 28-day survival parameter.

Design of in vivo study, which was described in the previous chapter, was selected as a model of endotoxicosis development that observed in suppurative peritonitis and destructive pancreatitis during postoperative period and always accompanied by severe toxemia due to the impossibility of immediate and complete elimination of its primary sources [1]. According to number of studies there are definite patterns in the movement of toxins by lymph and blood, no matter what's the nature of the primary site of endogenous intoxication (EI), status of detoxification and excretion of toxins systems, the nature of the underlying disease. At the initial stages of the EI development, toxins get into the blood generally by the lymph. By progressing of this process, most of toxins may enter the blood stream directly from the tissues due to increased transendothelial permeability of capillary wall and also be presented in the blood that leads to the rapid accumulation of toxins. Against this background, natural systems of detoxification and excretion of toxic products are activated in the body (liver, kidney) that explains the presence of significant postmortal changes in these organs. Thus, the presence of potentially high-toxic source of bacteria and/or their toxins that often presented in surgical endotoxicosis (unsanitary inflammation area or inflammation area without possibility of localization), leads to outstripping accumulation of toxins in the blood in comparison with the lymph (even if constant outer lymph efflux is organized) in a majority of cases. Therefore, only the overactive functioning of natural detoxification and elimination systems can inhibit further growth of toxemia. If patient was initially decompensated due to severe concomitant diseases, that determined liver or kidney failure (for example, cirrhosis or chronic renal failure), then toxicosis development against the background of SIRS will be even more dramatic. In this case, even relatively moderate concentration increase of concentration of toxins or other biologically active substances threaten rapid growth of multiple organ failure (MOF) symptoms. According to number of experts, the only effective solution is beginning of additional systemic detoxification before presenting of systemic organ failure symptoms. In these cases, the subject of detoxification is the blood, because there is elimination of toxins that was infiltrated into the systemic bloodstream. At the same time, the above-mentioned authors propose the "ideal" model of extracorporeal detoxification that suppose combination of lymph and blood detoxification, which can significantly reduce the development of systemic pathological changes in internal organs tissue due to impaired microcirculation and thus prevent the development of multiorgan failure. However, all authors worry about the lack of effectiveness of existing technologies for the separation and binding toxins and other pathognomonic biological active substances from biological media for the development of MODS.

The obtained data suggest triggers (microorganisms and their toxins) and inflammatory mediators (IL-6, IL- 10, IL-18) to secrete by immune cells and play an extremely role in the pathogenesis of SIRS and sepsis, so the impact on the stages of inflammation cascade should be regarded as an important component of complex approach in the treatment of septic complications. In particular, the obtained data from the studies on experimental animals with LPS-induced shock suggests that the prompt and, possibly, more effective elimination of bacterial endotoxins from the circulating blood is able to prevent unfolding of SIRS cascade or at least significantly reduce the severity of system pathological changes in the tissues of internal organs that was determined by impaired microcirculation. Therefore, it can prevent the development of organ and multiorgan failure, leading to the death. The accomplishment of management of the SIRS development and effective detoxification of the body by removal of exogenous antigens of various origins and endotoxins is realized by the use of different approaches of extracorporeal detoxification like measures of efferent therapy.

In the described prospective study of 97 cancer patients, in whom treatment was applied extracorporeal detoxification, there was analyzed correlation change of general condition of patients with change in laboratory parameters of patients' blood. The procedure of extracorporeal detoxification was carried out to 78 patients that were included in the study in the complex of intensive therapy in postoperative period; 45 patients weren't needed surgery and the use of extracorporeal detoxification was required for the chemotherapy complications relief of chemotherapy complications. From 1 to 4 procedures of ECD was carried out to each patient. The clinical efficacy of these procedures in the treatment of severe sepsis in cancer patients was assessed by vasopressor dose reduction, body temperature normalization, leucocytes concentration, procalcitonin and lactate levels (Table 3.1).

The result of carrying out HS and HDF procedures to patients with septic complications was a significant hyperthermia decrease. A similar trend was observed after the course of the HF, although it was not statistically confirmed. However, after HS procedure there was observed a statistically significant decrease in the blood concentration of PCT and decrease of dopamine and adrenaline doses needed to support the cardiovascular system and, which is likely to be regarded as an improvement of the clinical condition of the patients as a result of this procedure.

It is known that in extracorporeal detoxification there are used devices for the selective or nonselective hemosorption. Nowadays, for non-selective hemosorption, there are widely-used columns, containing modified granulated activated charcoal (Adsorba 300c or 150c, CytoSorb), and for selective hemosorption there are LPS-absorbers (Alteco, Toraymyxin).

At present study there were included 47 patients with lung (25), and gastrointestinal tract cancer (22) with severe sepsis that developed in the early postoperative period. There was carried out from 1 to 3 procedures of HS with the use of Adsorba 300c or Adsorba 150c, when the clinical signs of organ or organ failure were detected. If there was gram-negative sepsis evidence, then selective LPS-absorbers (Alteco) were used. Duration of each procedure was 2 hours. The effectiveness of the procedure was estimated by the changes in clinical and immunological parameters and also in the level change of bacterial endotoxin in the blood of patients.

The conducted studies showed that the application of LPS-adsorber decreased level of bacterial endotoxin (trigger factor in escalation of cytokine cascade) almost 3-fold in the blood serum of patients with sepsis (from 0.94 to 0.27 U/ml, $p<0.05$).

Moreover, a clear trend in the reduction of blood levels of IL-6, TNFα and IL-10 (mediators of systemic inflammatory reaction) was observed in most patients, although there was noted increase of cytokines after procedure in a number of patients in comparison with base level. Moreover, there were obtained data about concentration increase of soluble cytokine receptors in the blood after this procedure: level of sR IL-1 II was increased from 3.0 (2.5-3.2) pg/ml to 3.7 (3.0-3.8) pg/ml, $p=0.018$ and level of sR IL-6 - from 32.5 (29,7-37,8) pg/ml to 39,9 (28,7-42,4) pg/ml, $p=0.237$. Taking into account the possible hidden cytokinemia, we can assume that, due to contact with sorbent, there is dissociation of specific cytokine-receptor concentrations or non-specific cytokine-protein complexes by the gradient of concentration with the release of free cytokines, which can be detected by the applied test systems. This assumption was confirmed by the fact that there was detected high level of several cytokines (IL-4, IL-10, IL-6, IL-8) in eluates from sorbent of column after the procedure, while the identified cytokines receptors content was negligible. These LPS and cytokines level changes in blood of patients was accompanied by blood pressure normalization (51 ± 4,2 mm Hg to 62 ±

5,7 mm Hg, p=0.024), decrease of noradrenaline and dopamine infusions' rate (38,0 ± 3,4 against 10,2 ± 5,2 mg/min, p<0.01 and 16±3,3 against 8±2,9 μg/kg/min, p=0.014, respectively). There was also noted evident trend to level increase of hemoglobin saturation by oxygen (SpO2) and oxygenation index (PaO2/FiO2). The obtained data showed that use of LPS-adsorber resulted in a significant decrease of endotoxemia and cytokinemia, which correspond to the results of other researchers [2,3]. That suggests a hypothesis of existence of a cause-and-effect link between the removal of bacterial endotoxin from blood circulation and cytokines excess with positive changes in clinical status of patients with sepsis after hemoperfusion through LPS-adsorber.

Table 3.1. Changing the main clinical and laboratory parameters of the state of cancer patients with sepsis as a result of the HS, GDF, GF

Procedure	Parameters	Before procedure			After procedure			p
		Мед	25%	75%	Мед	25%	75%	
HS, n=67	Leukocytes, ×10^6 cells/ml	19	12	26	18	10	22	0.693
	Dopamine, μg/kg/min	6,0	4,2	9,0	4,0	0,0	6,0	0.025*
	Noradrenalin, μg/kg/min	10,00	3,00	17,00	8,50	0,56	14,00	0.240
	Adrenalin, μg/kg/min	7,0	1,4	17,0	0,0	0,0	11,0	0.034*
	T, °C	37,6	37,0	38,1	36,9	36,6	37,4	0.033*
	PCT, ng/ml	10,0	5,8	19,3	2,3	1,5	24,5	0.0002*
HDF, n=32	Leukocytes, ×10^6 cells/ml	23	21	27	24	21	27	0,668
	Dopamine, μg/kg/min	3,0	2,3	5,0	3,0	2,0	5,5	0,939
	Noradrenalin, μg/kg/min	0,50	0,16	1,00	0,55	0,14	1,00	0,871
	Adrenalin, μg/kg/min	2,0	1,0	2,0	3,5	1,0	3,5	0,361
	T, °C	37,8	37,4	38,4	37,3	36,9	37,6	0,009*
	PCT, ng/ml	27,0	10,0	48,0	80,0	17,0	85,6	0,462
HF, n=17	Leukocytes, ×10^6 cells/ml	17	10	24	16	16	24	0,805
	Dopamine, μg/kg/min	3,0	2,0	4,9	2,0	0,2	4,5	0,380
	Noradrenalin, μg/kg/min	70,0	60,0	80,0	75,0	50,0	100,0	0,687
	Adrenalin, μg/kg/min	37,3	37,0	38,0	36,8	36,6	36,9	0,079
	T, °C	69,0	3,0	102,0	69,0	4,0	77,0	0,874

*p<0.05.

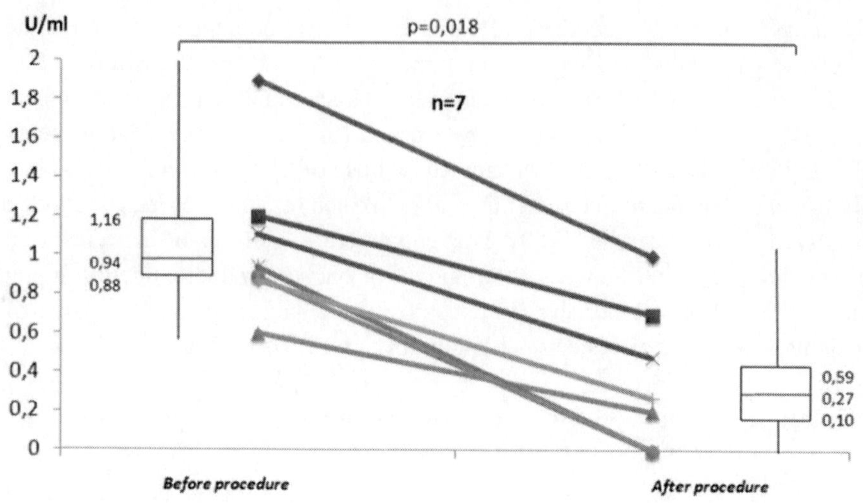

Figure 3.1.

Extracorporeal detoxification with the use of non-selective hemosorbents, which based on granular carbon sorbent is also led to body temperature normalization in patients with postoperative complications, reducing vasopressor load by dopamine (from 6,0 (4,2-9,0) µg/kg/min to 4.0 (0-0.6) µg/kg/min, p=0.025) and significant PCT reduction day after the procedure (10,0 (5,8-19,3) ng/ml to 2.3 (1,5-24,5) ng/ml, p=0.002). Although the statistical analysis did not confirm the significance of the changes in the studied parameters (p>0.05), but at the end of the procedure of HS, there was observed a significant decrease in serum levels of LPS (from 0,2 (0-1,92) IU/ml to 0.06 (0-0.92) IU/ml) and IL-18 (from 475(385-564) pg/ml to 331 (287-348) pg/ml). In the group of patients with based LPS level other than "0" there was a significant reduction of bacterial endotoxin after procedure with the Adsorba column (p=0.009). Furthermore, there were observed high endotoxin activity in the eluates from the sorbents after hemoperfusion that indicate about effective extraction of its free and plasma protein-bound forms by carbon sorbent. Although there were obtained data about multidirectional nature of the serum level changes of cytokines IL-6, IL-10, IL-18 as a result of the HS procedure, but in general, there was observed an obvious trend of a reduction of significant parameters on the background of their initial extremely high concentrations that resulted in normalization of functional activity of immunocompetent cells. In particular, there was observed decrease in NK-activity of blood ML of patients with sepsis from the values that exceeded the normal in 2,0-20,5 times (depending on the ratio of target cells and effector cells) to the level of healthy donors. Similarly, as a result of the phagocytic activity normalization of the neutrophils, there was observed downward trend of the PI and PF. The probable reasons of this effect can be reduction of co-stimulated molecules of cytokines (e.g. IL-8) in the blood flow and enhanced molecules shedding from the membranes of potential phagocytes that provide phagocytosed particles capturing. There were detected high concentrations of IL-6 and IL-18 in the washings from the sorbents. At the same time, there was noted significant increase in the concentration of cytokine receptor (s IL-1 II R – in 2.8 times, s TNF IR – in 1.7 times) after the procedure of HS. In addition, there were observed negligible level of LBP protein molecules, sCD14 and receptors to cytokines in eluates from sorbents. The increase of serum levels of soluble cytokine receptors may indicate to elimination of bound forms of cytokines during hemoperfusion due to the dissociation of the ligand-receptor complexes to free forms of cytokines and their receptors. It seems that released cytokines bind with the sorbent, while the soluble receptors are returned to the bloodstream and can inactivate inflammatory mediators.

Despite the fact that there was a concentration decrease of LPS and a number of endogenous bio-regulators in the blood after the procedure of HS, there was noted a trend for re-rising of these parameters in some patients a day after the procedure. Therefore, there is required a course of consistent procedures of HS in order to achieve sustainable effect. We analyzed the dynamics of LPS level, cytokines and their receptors in the blood serum of cancer patients with sepsis in the course which included 3 daily procedures of HS, using Adsorba 300c columns. The obtained data showed a significant reduction in serum levels of LPS in patients after the first procedure of HS. By the end of the third procedure there was observed stabile low, almost undetectable level of this analyte. These changes were accompanied by normalization of blood concentration of proinflammatory cytokines IL-1, IL-6 and TNFα of these patients as well as receptors to the corresponding cytokines that is likely to cause modulation of the level of blood neutrophils activation to normal levels: PI - from based 79% to 40% after the third procedure, and the PF - from 31 to 15 granules. That provided a significant decrease of release of "oxygen blow" products', neutrophils' type of free oxygen radicals, hydrogen peroxide, that are cytopathogenic for surrounding cells, and, first of all, for endotheliocytes.

CONCLUSION

The use for extracorporeal detoxification for cancer patients with sepsis both low-specific carbon hemosorbents and LPS-selective adsorbers followed by elimination of bacterial LPS and a wide range of cytokines from the blood circulation, as well as normalization of the effectors' functional activity of innate immunity that led to decrease in the severity of the patients (reduction of the required vasopressor support, serum level of PCT, normalization of body temperature, heart rate and blood pressure), which indicates to pathogenic validity of the application of pathogenetic hemosorption as a part of the complex treatment of sepsis and septic shock, particularly in the form of a course of consistently repetitive procedures. The results of the conducted studies suggest the following practical guidelines: extracorporeal detoxifycation should be started with the use of selective LPS-absorbers, if there is confirmed or suspected gram-negative sepsis; as a one-time procedure it is not always possible to achieve a stable effect, it is needed the course of consistent procedures under the control of the level of the triggers and inflammatory mediators in the systemic circulation; to improve the clinical efficacy of extracorporeal detoxification methods in sepsis, it should be applied in the early stages of the development of SIRS, before the onset of irreversible morphological changes in the target organs.

REFERENCES

[1]   Rozhkov, AG; Karandin, VI. Efferent therapy in the surgical clinic. Moscow. *Miklos*, 2010. 256 p.

[2]   Johnson, GB; Brunn, GJ; Platt, JL. Activation of mammalian Toll-like receptors by endogenous agonists. *Crit. Rev. Immunol*, 2003, 23, 15-44.

[3]   Robertson, CM; Coopersmith, CM. The systemic inflammatory response syndrome. *Microbes Infect*, 2006, 8(5), 1382-9.

In: Immunological Pathogenesis of Sepsis ...   ISBN: 978-1-62948-674-1
Editor: Natalia Yu. Anisimova   © 2014 Nova Science Publishers, Inc.

Chapter 4

DETOXIFICATION OF BLOOD AND PLASMA BY MEANS OF HYPERCROSSLINKED POLYMERIC HEMOSORBENTS: STATE-OF-THE-ART

V. A. Davankov[*], *M. P. Tsyurupa and L. A. Pavlova*

A.N. Nesmeyanov Institute of Organoelement Compounds, Russian Academy of Sciences, Vavilova St. 28, 119991, Moscow, Russian Federation

ABSTRACT

Extracorporeal blood detoxification by hemoperfusion is generally accepted to present the most efficient means for both a rapid removal of chemical toxins in cases of acute poisoning or drug overdoses and life-long support of patients on hemodialysis. More recently, in addition to traditional surface modified activated carbons, mesoporous polymeric adsorbing materials of a new generation, hypercrosslinked polymeric networks, have been found to be extremely effective in removing a whole palette of low-molecular-weight toxic proteins, cytokines, pro- and anti-inflammatory stimulators and mediators. This property of the material makes hemoperfusion an indispensable aid in combating acute inflammations and sepses.

---

[*] Corresponding author: Vadim A. Davankov Email: davank@ineos.ac.ru.

Present chapter provides first-hand information on principles of preparation of hypercrosslinked polymers, their structure and basic properties. Convincing proves for the unprecedented hemocompatibility of hypercrosslinked polydivinylbenzene and hypercrosslinked polystyrene are presented as well as results of their successful *in vitro* and *in vivo* tests and veterinary and clinical use. The polydivinylbenzene material CytoSorb has been approved in European Union as first-in-class cytokine extracorporeal filter in cytokine storm. The non-specific hypercrosslinked polystyrene-type sorbent Styrosorb was found to provide a complex removal of chemical toxins, numerous cytokines, lipopolysaccharides and blocking the proliferation of pathogenic bacterial cells and fungi. This material, too, is on its way to wide clinical applications.

1. EXTRACORPOREAL BLOOD PURIFICATION

Basic Information

Extracorporeal purification of blood is a medical procedure which is implemented outside the patient body and aimed at the removal of toxic compounds from its blood. The procedure may be divided into two main categories, hemoperfusion (hemosorption) and hemodialysis.

Hemoperfusion is a modern method of extracorporeal removing certain toxic compounds from blood or plasma of a patient by passing blood stream through a cartridge filled with a sorbent and then returning the thus treated blood to the body. Generally, one lets twice the whole blood circulating in the body to pass through the cartridge. Depending on the disease, doctor determines the type of the sorbent, its quantity, and the number of repeating treatment procedures. The method of hemoperfusion is intended to be used in both the cases of exogenous intoxications caused by numerous toxic chemicals and endogenous intoxications when tissue decay products or certain metabolites build up in blood of patients suffering from kidney or liver failure, hematite, pancreatitis, etc. Thus, hemoperfusion is extremely helpful in rapid treatment of acute poisoning through drug overdoses, narcotics, salts of heavy metals, or any other chemicals. Likewise, the procedure proves very efficient in treatment of autoimmune diseases, psoriasis, eczema, dermatitis, drug or food allergy, severe inflammations. Hemoperfusion was even shown to help patients suffering with some mental deceases.

Currently two basic types of sorbents for hemoperfusion are used in practice. The first type is presented by non-specific sorbents, largely activated carbons and, more recently, advanced polymeric sorbents. They extract from blood simultaneously many organic exogenic and endogenic compounds. The second type is composed of selective sorbents, such as ion exchange resins which are aimed at the removal of ammonium salts, excess potassium or phosphate ions, as well as heavy metals. Synthetic immunoaffine sorbents the structure of which incorporates special ligands capable of binding some specific toxic compounds, also relate to the second type of hemosorbents.

Sorbents for extracorporeal blood purification should meet three principal requirements. In the first place, they must effectively extract target compounds from whole blood or plasma, second, they must be hemocompatible, and third, they must be mechanically stable and not contain particulates or produce fines during hemoperfusion procedures, which would cause embolism of capillary blood vessels.

Efficiency of hemosorbents is determined by the whole complex of structural and chemical features of the material, such as mean pore diameter and pore size distribution, specific surface area accessible to the target toxicant, chemical nature of the surface and its functional groups, including biospecific ligands. These properties are responsible for both the kinetics of mass transfer within the sorbent bead and strength of binding of toxicants to the surface or its functional groups.

The term "hemocompatible" means that a sorbent, which immediately contacts blood stream, does not release any alien chemical components, cause any change in blood cell corpuscles, activate clotting cascade or have an undesired influence on blood composition, e.g., extract inadmissibly large amount of albumin or other essential blood components. It is appropriate to note here that another term "biocompatibility" is often found in the literature. It means the ability of a material, after being implanted in patient's tissue or organs, to remain in the organism without causing collateral clinical displays, while still performing the required mechanical function and inducing necessary cellular or tissue responses which are needed to achieve an optimal therapeutic effect. The notion "hemocompatible material" unambiguously tells about the passivity of the material with respect to blood, while "biocompatible material" is not necessarily inert towards blood. In addition to aforementioned basic requirements, one has to point out that both hemosorbents and biocompatible implant materials must tolerate appropriate sterilization procedures and retain all their useful properties.

The development of materials characterized by true hemocompatibility, in particular thromboresistance, represents a complex problem. It should be said hear that in human body the surface of healthy blood vessels possesses antithrombotic properties since the membranes of epithelia cells contain heparin-like compounds with high concentration of sulfonate groups. Besides, the domain-type hydrophilic/hydrophobic structures of a blood vessel surface, which is similar to that characterizing circulatory blood, also play a specific role. Moreover, some biologically active substances, such as prostacyclin, nitrogen oxide, etc., come out in blood thus inhibiting the activation of platelets. Hence, in a healthy organism, the natural balance between the systems of activation and inhibition of fibrillation emerges on the boundary blood/internal vessel surface.

Immediate contact of circulating blood with a surface of foreign body, for instance, with that of activated carbon-type sorbent, shifts the above equilibrium and results in the activation of clotting cascade due to the activation of internal fibrillation system, and adhesion of platelets on the sorbent.

In order to preclude extremely undesirable consequences of clotting during hemoperfusion, a large dose of an antithrombotic preparation, heparin, is usually injected in blood stream. However, its application may be accompanied with serious by-effects. Heparin generally influences the metabolism of lipids and bone tissue. Not all patients tolerate heparin well. Especially dangerous is internal bleeding, particularly, if a patient suffers from stomach or intestines ulcer. In the event that strong internal bleeding happened, hemoperfusion procedure has to be discontinued and the bleeding has to be stopped by injection of heparin antagonist, protamine-sulfate. Unfortunately, the latter itself is a toxic compound and causes many serious by-effects. Consequently, the blood heparinisation, though being inevitable during hemosorption on activated carbons, still is a quite undesirable procedure.

A usual way of imparting sorbents hemocompatibility consists in the chemical modification of their surface. This modification may be realized by different methods which we will discuss in the following separately for each type of hemosorbents.

In fact, hemoperfusion is known for a long time. The first attempt to remove urea from blood of uremic patients by adsorption on sorbents was made as far back as 1948 [1]. Carbon was shown to eliminate some particular components from the blood, such as creatinine, uric acid, guanidine, indoles, phenolic compounds and organic acids [2]. At the same time, adsorption of urea was insufficient. Besides, hemoperfusion does not solve another even more acute problem of uremic patients, which is removing excess water. This problem is only resolved by applying another procedure, hemodialysis.

Hemodialysis is the common modern way of supporting life in the case of renal failure. By letting blood to equilibrate with a special dialysate aqueous solution across a semipermeable polymeric membrane, hemodialysis allows both the excess water and small molecules like urea to migrate down the pressure and concentration gradients from the blood into the dialysate fluid. The introduction of hemodialysis into medical practice extends the life expectancy of patients with end-stage renal disease (ESRD) for about 5 years on an average.

The first devices of hemodialysis utilized natural cellulose (cuprophan) membranes which possessed predominantly small pores. These membranes were capable of removing excess fluid containing ions and small molecules with molecular weight less than approximately 1,200 Dalton. Later, the development of new synthetic polysulfone or polyacrylonitrile dialysis membranes that possessed larger pores and, in combination with equipment to better control transmembrane pressure, permitted more efficient elimination of middle molecules, in addition to small ones. These high-flux hollow fiber membranes came into routine practice after appearing in 1985 the investigation results of Gcyjo et al. [3] who established the link between the accumulation of B_2-microglobulin (B_2M) in the body of uremia patients and complications caused by long-term dialysis (called Dialysis-Related Amyloidosis, DRA). As kidney failure progresses, β_2M concentration in the extracellular compartments increases, often by a factor of 30 to 60. In the DRA complication, insoluble plaques of β_2M and its glycosilation products (known as amyloid fibrils) gradually accumulate in joints causing a huge pain, progressive crippling arthritis, inflammatory arthropathy of the joints and spine. Patients with DRA often require surgery to correct carpal tunnel syndrome, a common manifestation of DRA, and lifelong medications to ameliorate joint pain and inflammation. Several investigators have shown that the partial removal of β_2M with high-flux membranes retards, but not prevents, the onset of DRA in dialysis patients.

Hemodialysis procedure has to be repeated three or four times a week. This is a slow process, which keeps the patient connected to the stationary dialysis machine for several hours. Beside the high consumption of the expensive apyrogenic physiological dialysate fluid (about 120 L), the technique is unpleasant and inconvenient for the patient. The patient feels unwell both before and after dialysis. Before dialysis the waste products build up in the body, and after dialysis there is a dramatic distortion of the balance of chemical equilibria and processes in the body due to the rapid removal of about 3 L water and a whole pool of molecules of the molecular weight below

500 Da. Among these molecules are all essential amino acids, nucleotides, some mineral ions and many other useful components.

Fresh high-flux membranes were found to reduce the level of B_2-microglobulin in plasma by 23-37 % [4]. Unfortunately, the reuse of rather expensive membranes significantly deteriorates the extent of the target protein removal [5]. It was recognized that the removal of B_2M is conditioned upon the adsorption of middle molecules on the surface of the high-flux membrane rather than their diffusion through the membrane [6, 7]. With the surface area of membranes in the dialysis device amounting to less than 2 m^2, the adsorption capacity of the device is obviously too small and gets used up during the first dialysis session.

Much more efficient in removing B_2M should be the use of adsorbing materials, e.g. activated carbons, since specific surface area of these materials easily approaches 1000-2000 m^2/g and a hemoperfusion device can easily incorporate several hundred grams of the adsorbent. However, activated carbons are not hemocompatible and cause coagulation of blood. Besides, activated carbons are not resistant to attrition, and, by releasing fins, cause embolism of blood capillaries. Recent review [8] of the use of sorbent hemoperfusion in end-stage renal decease describes manifold attempts to eliminate the above problems by introducing microencapsulation technique [9] by which the activated charcoal particles were coated with a polymer membrane, such as cellulose nitrate (collodin), cellulose acetate, methacrylic hydrogel, or crosslinked albumin. Unfortunately, every coating membrane creates significant diffusion barriers to larger toxic molecules and dramatically slows down their sorption kinetics, while not preventing the loss of many biologically important smaller molecules like amino acids, glucose, hormones, calcium, etc. [10] Though hemoperfusion on coated carbons reduces concentration of B_2M and toxic middle molecules, the undesired losses of fibrinogen, fibronectin, platelets, leucocytes and complement activation are also observed [11].

A special polymeric adsorbing material (BM-01, Kaneka, Japan) has been described by Japanese group [12] for the selective removal of β_2M from the blood of dialysis patients. The adsorbent consists of porous cellulose beads modified with hexadecyl groups that retain β_2M through hydrophobic interactions. The adsorption capacity of this material is 1 mg of β_2M per 1 mL of adsorbent. Using a hemoperfusion cartridge containing 350 mL of these cellulose beads in sequence with a high-flux hemodialyzer, several small clinical trials were performed. During 4 to 5 hours of treatment, about 210 mg of β_2M were removed, thus reducing its concentration in the blood by 60-70 %

of initial levels [13]. Clinical improvement was partial, but marked in those patients subjected to thrice weekly treatment with this device for a period of two months or more. Subjective improvements were seen in joint mobility, joint pain, and nocturnal awakening. The use of this device is currently restricted to Japan, and concerns over its high cost have largely prevented more widespread use [14].

At present there are over 350,000 patients treated for chronic kidney failure in the USA and nearly one million worldwide. These numbers increase by about 6 % every year. Though Medicare (the federal program in the USA of concessionary medical insurance for patients over 65 with severe kidney failure) spends annually about $45,000 US per patient, the morbidity and mortality statistics for this patient population is horrendous. Between 23 and 25 % of the US dialysis population die each year, and the average patient spends up to 16 days in the hospital each year being treated for serious, often life-threatening complications.

Thus, it is quite evident that medicine is in extreme need of a new cost-effective, selective, and high capacity adsorbent for the removal of middle-molecule toxic compounds and, first of all, β_2-microglobulin from blood or plasma. No wonder that many different suggestions appeared during the last decades, mainly described in patent literature, to prepare porous hemocompatible polymers which could be useful in supporting patients with renal failure.

2. REVIEW OF PATENT LITERATURE RELATED TO POLYMERIC HEMOSORBENTS

2.1. Removal of Toxins Related to Kidney Failure

Blood is a very complex biological liquid. Among the variety of proteins comprising the blood of healthy man there is a small relatively hydrophobic globular protein with molecular weight of 11.8 kDa, β_2-microglobulin (the protein of surface antigens of nucleated cells). If one assumes the spherical shape of its molecule, its diameter will amount to 3.35 nm. The concentration of the protein is pretty small, about 600 ng/mL, and rather constant. However, when the normal filtration function of kidney is disrupted the concentration of β_2-microglobulin in blood significantly rises. Hemodialysis, which renal chronics have to use, removes excess water and urea but fails to remove $\beta_2 M$.

The molecular size of this toxic protein is too large to come through dialysis membrane while the increase in size of the membrane pores would involve an inadmissible loss of albumin and other valuable proteins.

Hemosorption is the only way to selectively remove B_2-microglobulin from the blood of uremic patients. In overwhelming majority of cases one has employed activated carbon the surface of which was covered with a film of hemocompatible polymers. This modification, however, drastically slows down the diffusion of B_2M though the coating and deteriorates the sorption kinetics on carbons, generally good adsorbing materials. This fundamentally unavoidable shortcoming delayed the progress in the development of new hemosorbents based on activated carbons and the number of patent applications dropped. At the same time, the interest to polymeric adsorbents increased, because their porous structure may be easer adjusted to a desired value and their surface may be easier made hemocompatible.

In 1997 Davankov at al. [15, 16] suggested hypercrosslinked polystyrene adsorbing materials for the removal of B_2-microglobulin. The polymers of this type have been obtained [17] by an intensive crosslinking the chains of linear polystyrene in solution or in swollen state with bifunctional reagents, for instance, monochlorodimethyl ether. At first, the reagent introduces chloromethyl groups into phenyl rings of the initial polystyrene chains. (Obviously, one can introduce chloromethyl groups by any other appropriate method). Then, these reactive groups alkylate neighboring phenyl rings thus connecting them with methylene bridges. Due to the presence of a solvent (called porogen), this intensive crosslinking results in the formation of a rigid highly porous open-network-type structure. The surface-exposed chloromethyl groups fail to find a reactive partner to convert into an interchain crosslinking bridge and remain pendant. These groups are highly reactive and may be used for an appropriate modification of beads and pore surface by various compounds that improve hemocompatibility of the material. For example, it is possible to chemically bind heparin to the surface of particles. Another option is the electrostatic adsorption of heparin that has negatively charged sulfonate groups on the surface of beads preliminary modified with positively charged ionogenic groups. By using chloromethyl groups it is also possible to graft various hydrophilic polymeric chains which will prevent platelets from adsorption on the surface of the hydrophobic hypercrosslinked polystyrene beads. Still easier is substituting the surface chloromethyl groups with hydrophilic functional groups or residues of amino acids. These methods of surface chemical modification with the low molecular weight substances enhance the hydrophilicity and hemocompatibility of beads without putting obstacles for the diffusion of B_2-microglobulin into the interior of sorbent beads. Indeed, further studies demonstrated splendid hemocompatibility of the modified hypercrosslinked polystyrene sorbents and their ability to extract effectively toxic protein molecules.

Soon after appearing the above-mentioned publications of Davankov et al. [15, 16] several researches took up the idea of removing B_2M by means of various polymeric adsorbents, including conventional macroporous styrene-divinylbenzene copolymers, especially in view of an earlier (1992) report of the same group [18] showing that special types of these polymers may exhibit typical properties of hypercrosslinked polystyrene. Strom et al. [19-22] described the synthesis of conventional macroporous copolymers of divinylbenzene with 40 %, 20 % and 10 % ethyl styrene, as well as methods of imparting copolymer beads hemocompatibility. The authors proposed grafting hydrophilic polymers on the copolymer bead surface by involving pendant double bonds which, similar to chloromethyl groups of hypercrosslinked polystyrenes, mainly remain on the surface where they failed to find a partner during the initial polymerization process. The list of grafted polymers includes poly(alkylene glycol), poly(alkylphosphazene), polyvinylpyridines, poly-vinylimidazoles, poly(N-vinyl-2-pyrrolidone), polyacrylic and polymath-acrylic acids and their derivatives, such as poly(2-hydroxyethylmethacrylate), and even heparin. The main point of the above patents is that the grafting procedure consists in that the dried macroporous divinylbenzene copolymer is placed into methanolic solutions of the vinyl monomers and the initiator of free radical polymerization. In boiling methanol media, only surface double bonds of the copolymer are activated and involved into polymerization of added monomers. A serious drawback of suggested grafting hemocompatible polymer chains onto the surface of beads and that of macropores is that any polymer coating unavoidably reduces the diffusion rate of protein molecules to the hydrophobic surface where actually the sorption event must take place.

Another group of followers under the guidance of Albright [23] put in a claim for the patent defense the preparation of trivial macroporous copolymers of styrene with several polyfunctional monomers (divinylbenzene, trivinyl-benzene, trivinylcyclohexane, divinylnaphthalene, divinylsulfone, etc.) by the well-known suspension polymerization method, followed by radical grafting chains of poly(N-vinyl-2-pyrrolodone), poly(vinyl alcohol), polymethacrylic and polyacrylic acids, etc. The copolymers were reported to possess pores in the range between 100 and 300 E in diameter. They are not accessible to substances with molecular weights exceeding 50,000 Da, but readily adsorb compounds with molecular weights of less than 35,000 Da. The patent states that the porous polymers take up 90 % Cytochrome C, the model compound for B_2-microglobulin, and only 8-11 % albumin from an aqueous solution with pH 7.4-8.7.

Davankov et al. [24] proposed later a fundamentally new approach to the outer surface modification of copolymer beads aimed at the extracorporeal blood detoxification. Porous styrene copolymers are usually obtained by free radical copolymerization of comonomers dissolved in water-immiscible inert diluents, the organic phase being dispersed in the form of spherical droplets in an aqueous phase. While the generally accepted approach comprises the modification of synthesized and isolated copolymer beads, this patent suggests a one-pot modification of the beads without their isolation from the aqueous reaction medium. For this purpose, after completing the polymerization (or during polymerization) one adds into the aqueous phase a suitable water-soluble initiator of radical polymerization and then a water soluble monomer, for instance, N-vinyl-2-pyrrolidone. The latter reacts with double bonds that are predominantly activated on the surface of beads dispersed in the aqueous phase. As a result, short linear chains of the hydrophilic polymer form on the bead surface, rather than within their macropores. The latter retain their hydrophobic nature which is important for the sorption of toxins. Certainly, several other hydrophilic polymers possessing good hemocompatibility can be grafted to the surface by this technique. Numerous experiments carried out both *in vitro* and *in vivo* with hypercrosslinked polydivinylbenzene modified by poly(N-vinyl-2-pyrrolidone) using the above approach, demonstrated excellent hemocompatibility of the material. It is this material that served as the basic hemosorbent for subsequent numerous laboratory and clinical tests which will be described later in this chapter.

Beside B_2-microglobulin, other deleterious protein molecules, chemokines, that are a variety of cytokines (see below) were found to accumulate in the body of patients with kidney failure. Many chemokines represent pro-inflammatory cytokines stimulating the migration of immune cells to the nidus of infection. To remove chemokines together with B_2M from the blood of uremic patients Nanko et al. [25, 26] suggest a porous cellulose sorbent modified with hydrophobic organic molecules having 8 to 18 carbon atoms and characterized by log P>2.5 (where P is the distribution coefficient of the compound in standard octanol-water system). For example, the authors propose treating the cellulose beads with sodium hydroxide, then epichloro-hydrine and finally with hexadecylamine. Such sorbent extracts well B_2-microglobulin from human blood diminishing its concentration from 34.9 mg/L to7.7 mg/L during a four hour contact of the blood with the sorbent.

2.2. Removal of Toxins Related to Sepsis

Sepsis is a severe inflammatory condition of human body or animals resulting from a blood infection. More frequently, it appears as a consequence of surgery, trauma, suppurative inflammation, burn injury, etc. Inflammatory response is regulated by complex interactions of pro-inflammatory and anti-inflammatory stimulators and mediators. Known representatives of these compounds include, but are by no means limited to, cytokines, nitric oxide, thromboxanes, leukotrienes, platelet-activating factor, prostaglandins, kinins, complement factors, superantigens, monokines, chemokines, interferons, free radicals, proteases, arachidonic acid metabolites, prostacyclins, beta endorphins, myocardial depressant factors, anandamide, 2-arachidonoyl-glycerol, tetrahydrobiopterin, and chemicals including histamine, bradykinin, and serotonin.

The inflammatory response, when regulated and localized, is beneficial. However, if not regulated and generalized, the inflammatory response can cause significant tissue injury and even death.

Above mentioned cytokines present a whole class of proteins produced by macrophages, monocytes, and lymphocytes in response to viral or bacterial infection, as well as in response to T cell stimulation during an immune response. Cytokines possess a wide spectrum of immunological and non-immunological activities. They affect diverse physiologic functions, such as cell growth, differentiation, homeostasis and pathological physiology. Cytokines are also known to be capable of stimulating their own synthesis, as well as the production of other cytokines from a variety of cell types. This phenomenon is called the "cytokine cascade."

Cytokines are normally present in very low concentrations in the blood or tissues. However, the function of cytokine production can become disordered, e.g. in the case of severe inflammation or sepsis. Only one or a few initiating stimuli activate a variety of mediators. The concentration of cytokines raises leading to a rapid dissemination and extension of a great number of responses. As a result it can lead to the destruction of healthy organ tissues, multiple organ failure and even death. Therefore, if the sepsis is in progress while a medicamentous therapy fails to prevent the misbalance of many human functions the removal of toxins, first of all, cytokines, from blood of patients with sepsis via hemoperfusion seems to be the most promising approach.

Cytokines are proteins with molecular weight of 8,000 to 28,000 Da. That is why Brady, Davankov et al. [27-30] proposed cytokines removal from blood or plasma by means of non-specific porous polymeric adsorbing materials having pores of 2 to 7 nm in diameter. Most promising seems to be polymers belonging to the family of hypercrosslinked aromatic polymers. They can be obtained by intensive crosslinking of swollen beaded styrene-divinylbenzene copolymers with monochlorodimethyl ether or *p*-xylylene dichloride. Another way of preparing hypercrosslinked polystyrene-type sorbents consists in preliminary chloromethylation of a styrene-divinylbenzene copolymer followed by chains bridging in an organic solvent. Besides, required material may represent mesoporous styrene-divinylbenzene copolymers.

To impart the above hypercrosslinked hydrophobic polystyrene hemocompatibility the surface of spherical beads was suggested to treat as follows:

- to treat the residual chloromethyl groups of hypercrosslinked polystyrene with 2-ethanolamine and then to bind heparin at the expense of electrostatic forces;
- to substitute chloromethyl groups with 2-ethanolamine and bind heparin covalently by means of glutardialdehyde or hexamethyl-enediisocyanate, an then deactivate excess aldehyde or isocyanate groups by reaction with L-aspartic acid;
- to substitute chloromethyl groups with 2-ethanolamine or ethylene glycol, activate these ligands with glutardialdehyde or hexamethyl-enediisocyanate and then bind covalently hydrophilic chains of polyethylene glycol;
- to bind covalently hydrophilic chains of polyethylene glycol to the residual chloromethyl groups of the polymer using polyethylene glycol in the form of sodium alcoholate;
- to bind covalently hydrophilic chains of chitosan through the reaction of its amine groups with chloromethyl groups of the polymer;
- to substitute chloromethyl groups with 2-ethanolamine or ethylene glycol, react these ligands with phosphorous-oxychloride and then bind covalently choline, serine or 2-ethanolamine.

The polymers thus modified do not stimulate the production of cytokines and other pro- and anti-inflammatory stimulators and mediators, on the contrary, the polymers extract them from blood. The proposed adsorbing materials can be used in the cases when it is necessary to preclude, control, decrease or ease the gravity of inflammatory response of human body to diseases.

Sepsis may be caused by the presence in blood of pathogenic micro-organisms (bacteria, fungi). A medicamentous treatment of infected patients inevitably involves the emergence in blood of various low molecular weight (4,100-30,000) cyclic and acyclic organic compounds, such as acridines, dyes, psoralen and its derivatives, etc. Many of them while inactivating pathogenic microorganisms are toxic and, in their turn, have to be finally removed from blood or plasma. For this purpose Hei [31-34] proposed using a composite material composed of spherical particles of a porous polymeric adsorbent immobilized in a fibrous polymeric matrix. Various fiber-forming polymers (polyethylene, polyethylene terephthalate, polyamide, polyvinyl alcohol, polysulfone) were taken as the matrix. The fibers were rapidly heated till a high temperature (at which they started to melt) and mixed with a beaded sorbent. As the porous sorbent, the authors proposed the use of macroporous styrene-divinylbenzene copolymers Amberlite XAD-2, XAD-4, XAD-16, XAD-1180, as well as hypercrosslinked polystyrene sorbents XUS-43493 and MN-200 (manufactured by Dow Chemical Co and Purolite International Co, respectively). To make the adsorbents hemocompatible, their surface was modified with poly(hydroxymethylmethacrylate), polyethylene glycol or polyethyleneoxide. These polymeric modifying agents were applied to the bead surface either by adsorption from a solution or by sputtering the solution onto the surface of beads suspended in flow of air. The material thus obtained was then placed into a cartridge.

In the author's judgment, steam sterilization of the composite adsorbents is more reasonable than ε-irradiation. However, it was noted that the treatment with steam of water-saturated macroporous beads results in their partial shrinkage and noticeable loss of pores. Therefore, the author suggests soaking the sorbents with non-volatile polyethylene glycol (300 or 400 Da) or glycerol prior to heating (glycerol is hemocompatible; it is sometimes added to blood to prevent its freezing when storing at low temperature). As a whole, obtaining of the above composite material including the stage of its sterilization presents a rather complex and expensive process. Still, Hei claims that the developed composite material may remove cytokines, in addition to drugs applied to sepsis patients.

Nakamura et al. [35] claims that one may obtain a biocompatible polymer capable of removing endotoxins and other pathogenic components from blood, if one makes a porous polymer that is hydrophilic on the bead surface and rater hydrophobic in the pore interior. The starting material is a macroporous styrene-divinylbenzene copolymer prepared by free radical polymerization of comonomers dissolved in a mixture of two porogens, toluene and isoamyl alcohol. The former solvent is known to be responsible for the formation of small pores in the final polymer while isoamyl alcohol makes very large pores, up to several microns in size. The polymer was subjected to chloromethylation, dried and treated with an aqueous solution of polyethylene glycol (ca 1,000 Da). The chloromethylated copolymer is hydrophobic and does not swell in water, so that only the outer surface-exposed chloromethyl groups of polymer beads convert into hydrophilic and hemocompatible functions. Those chloromethyl groups residing on the internal pore surface were then transformed to amine groups, carboxylic groups or epoxy functions by appropriate reactions in organic solvents. The internal surface of final beads is responsible for the sorption properties of the material. The latter takes up 16-45 mg/g heparin.

A device for the treatment of animals suffering from chronic diseases and acute inflammatory processes was proposed in [36, 37]. The device comprises a hemofilter and an adsorption column. The hemofilter is aimed at the obtaining of two blood streams, namely, plasma and blood stream enriched with cells. Inflammatory mediators are removed from the plasma stream by adsorption on a sorbent. A therapeutic agent is added to the purified plasma and then the latter is mixed with the stream enriched with cells and both return in the animal body. Since the device makes provision for the contact of sorbents with plasma stream, rather than whole blood stream, many different adsorbing materials can be applied. Silica gel, activated carbon, ion exchange resins, neutral polymers, cellulose and its esters, polysulfone, polyacrylamide, polymethylmethacrylate, polyamide, polycarbonate, polystyrene-based fibers, immobilized polymyxin B, monoclonal antibodies, immobilized specific antagonists, etc. were suggested on the list of sorbents for the removal of inflammatory toxins.

2.3. Removal of Toxins Related to Liver Failure

Acute liver failure or severe damage of the liver caused by different etiologies, including sepsis, involves complex mechanisms resulting in severe disturbances of principle liver detoxification functions followed by accumulation of hydrophobic toxic metabolites in the blood. However, metabolites such as bile acids, bilirubin, tryptophan, and phenolic compounds are albumin-bound and therefore, they cannot be removed by hemodialysis [38]. Thus, bilirubin is strongly albumin-bound with an association constant of $9.5\cdot10^7$ M^{-1}, corresponding to an unbound fraction at the equilibrium of less than 0.1 %, while the free fraction of weaker bound cholic acid amounts to about 16 %. In order to compensate the liver's missing function as efficiently as possible, strong adsorptive techniques are required for depletion of such toxins. The problem with hemocompatibility of strong hydrophobic adsorbing materials becomes especially actual.

Roberts and Litzie [39] have patented a device for removing toxins from blood of patients with liver affected by sepsis. The device comprises a system for separating blood cells from plasma, the removal of toxins from plasma by adsorption onto a mixture of sorbents, and returning both plasma and blood corpuscles back to the patient blood stream. The system is much more complicated than a simple cartridge used in direct hemoperfusion, but avoids the problems with hemocompatibility of sorbents. Such materials can be applied as unmodified activated carbons of different origin, commercial ion exchange resin Amberlite XAD-7 HP, neutral aliphatic polyester resins with specific surface area of 500 m^2/g and average pore diameter of 45 nm, or commercial macroporous styrene-divinylbenzene resin Amberchrom CG300-C having surface area of 600-700 m^2/g and average pore size of 30 nm. (A more detailed study with neutral polystyrene-divinylbenzene resins [40] showed that only pores larger than 5-6 nm were accessible to strongly albumin-bound substances, such as bilirubin. On the other hand, less strongly albumin-bound substances, such as bile acids, were better removed by polymers of the small pore size range).

In *in vitro* experiments the plasma of human blood spiked with 20 mg/dL bilirubin, 5 mg/dL creatinine and 20 mg/dL urea was circulated within six hours through 36 g activated carbon, 31 g XAD-7 or Amberchrom. The first adsorbent reduced the level of bilirubin, urea and creatinine by 49.5 %, 24.7 % and 97.9 %, respectively. XAD-7 extracted 34.6 % bilirubin, 11.2 % urea and 9.0 % creatinine. Amberchrom removed 95.7 % bilirubin, 11.2 % urea and 10.1 % creatinine. Unfortunately, the sorbents also extracted 15-20 % albumin and other proteins. In another *in vitro* experiment a cartridge was packed with the mixture of 100 g activated carbon, 35 g XAD-7 and 35 g Amberchrom. Heparinized plasma containing 20, 50 and 15 mg/dL bilirubin, urea and creatinine, respectively, was percolated through the cartridge. This mixture of sorbents removed 41.4 % bilirubin, 30.7 % urea and 78.3 % creatinine. Beside these endogenic toxins the plasma was spiked with 75-200 mg/mL acetaminophen, the concentration of which dropped by 82.4 % after completing the session. The loss of albumin and total proteins was 10-15 % while the loss of fibrinogen amounted to 25-30 %. Though providing an idea about the selectivity of the above three adsorbents, these results are considered to be inconclusive because the volume of circulating plasma was not specified.

Testing of the above plasma perfusion device in *in vivo* experiments with eight dogs showed its safety; no leucopenia and thrombocytopenia were observed. The comparison of blood parameters before and after inserting the device in plasma circuit demonstrated that the change in electrolytic balance and the adsorption of fibrillation factors do not occur. At the same time, it was noted that for four hour plasma sorption the arterial blood pressure of dogs rose.

In order to facilitate the adsorption kinetics of albumin-bound hydrophobic metabolites related to liver failure (bilirubin, cholic acid), as well as cytokines (TNF-α, IL-6), using of microparticulate polystyrene-divinylbenzene resins was suggested. The average size of particles was about 50 μm, average pore size of the microparticles was 7.7 nm and the BET surface was 680 m^2/g. The particles must be imbedded into a cryogel of polyvinylalcohol or agarose, though the imbedding procedure negatively affects both the adsorption capacity of the composite and rates of adsorption of the toxins from blood plasma [41].

By using efficient membranes that separate plasma circuit from blood, particle size of sorbents can be reduced to diameters as small as 1–10 μm. The particles are circulating in plasma suspension. The safety of the system is guaranteed by the use of fluorescently labeled magnetic microparticles, which in case of a membrane-leakage are detected in the blood circuit by an optical system equipped with a magnetic trap. The extracorporeal liver support system was successfully tested in *in vitro* experiments with blood spiced with unconjugated bilirubin and cholic acid to 300 μmol/L and 100 μmol/L, respectively [42].

Leistner and Leistner [43] proposed using copolymers of 1-vinylimidazole or 1-vinyl-2-methylimidazole with divinylbenzene for the removal from blood or plasma of medicinal albumin-bound preparations, in addition to exogenic and endogenic toxins. The polymer was prepared by radical copolymerization of the comonomers in the presence of inert diluents (such as toluene, 1,2-dichloroethane, carbon tetrachloride, ethyl acetate, butyl acetate). The diluents were used individually or as a mixture. The spherical macroporous polymer beads are characterized by specific surface area of 900 m^2/g, total pore volume of 2 cm^3/g, and average pore diameters varying from 100 to 500 E. The polymers rapidly absorb low molecular weight compounds as N-acetyltryptophan, phenol, fatty acids, caffeine, albumin-bound toxins and bilirubin. The authors claim the polymers to exhibit good hemocompatibility confirmed by citotoxicologic and hemolysis tests.

In his patent of 2003 Hei [34] also mentioned the removal of psoralen as well as its photo degradation products from plasma depleted with platelets of patients with hepatitis. Psoralen is a tricyclic compound comprising structural fragments of furan and coumarin. Psoralen is known to inactivate the hepatitis virus; however, it is capable of building-in between the DNA helixes disturbing its basic function. To extract the toxic drug Hei suggests macroporous sorbents Amberlite XAD-2, XAD-4, XAD-16, XAD-2000, activated carbons, silica gels and hypercrosslinked polystyrene Dowex XUS 43943, all modified at the surface by 2-hydroxymethylmetactylate. The sorbents reduce the psoralen concentration to 1 mM.

Eguchi et al. [44] described equipment for obtaining monosized particles of porous polymeric hemosorbents using a well-known principle of jetting. Briefly, one prepares a fine emulsion of a rather viscous polymer (polymers) solution in an appropriate immiscible liquid and lets the emulsion to pass through vibrating extrusion nozzles into a bath with a coagulating liquid where the process of crosslinked polymer formation is completed. The process permits obtaining uniformly sized particles (having the diameter no less than 80 мм and no more that 300 мм) of styrene copolymers, polyvinyl alcohol, cellulose, silk, collagen, etc. To evaluate whether or not the resulting polymers are suitable for the extracorporeal blood purification, particles of cellulosc acetate were packed in column of 7 mm in diameter and 10 mm in length. Bovine blood diluted with 3 % solution of anticoagulant, sodium citrate, in tris-buffer (9:1 by volume) was sent through the column. Although the pressure drop across the column steadily rose (in one hour contact time it amounted to 85 mm Hg) the authors believe these data to be acceptable and testify to the absence of hemolysis.

Inorganic microporous ion exchange silica materials containing zirconium or titanium were suggested in [45, 46]. The product was obtained, for example, by heating an aqueous mixture of colloidal silica with KOH and zirconium acetate at 200 °C for 36 hours. The material is capable of exchanging potassium ions for NH_4^+ ions which are present in blood or in dialysis liquid after the hemodialysis session.

2.4. Brief Evaluation of the Patent Literature

Analysis of the above patents permits drawing an unambiguous conclusion that the source materials have not enough information. There authors pretend to protect a maximum possible number of synthesis protocols and polymeric hemosorption products without indicating the optimal variant and presenting sufficient results of real use of the hemosorbents in *in vitro* or *in vivo* experiments. Nevertheless, it is possible to draw some general conclusions about the modern trends in hemosorption technology.

Importantly, during the last two decades the interest of researches to activated carbons went down. Although up to now in the practice of hemosorption, active carbon still presents the dominating type of sorbent, its negative properties have become very evident. Above all, activated carbon is incompatible with whole blood and unavoidably leads to thrombosis. To preclude this quite undesirable consequence, it is necessary both to modify sorbent surface and introduce in the blood stream special anticoagulants. Heparin is the most widespread anticoagulant of natural origin. However, its application may be accompanied by serious hemorrhages, especially if a patient has ulcer of stomach. Formation of a hydrophilic polymeric membrane on the surface of carbon particles improves its hemocompatibility, but inevitable impairs kinetics of sorption and deteriorates the adsorption capacity towards relatively large toxic molecules. Also, low mechanical and attrition strengths of activated carbon leads to release of fine particulates.

Therefore, new developments are aimed at the use of hemocompatible polymeric sorbents displaying high affinity to both low molecular weight chemicals and a broad spectrum of middle molecular toxic proteins. Most promising non-specific sorbents proved to be macroporous copolymers of divinylbenzene with styrene, acrylic and methacrylic acid esters. Majority of researchers give preference to styrene-divinylbenzene copolymers. It is conditioned upon the circumstance that all factors determining the formation of their porous structure have been studied in detail. Therefore, the synthesis of a mechanically resistant polymeric matrix having express adsorption potential, particle size and porous structure one needs for a future hemosorbent, now is no more than a technical problem.

Providing the polystyrenic matrix with the property of hemocompatibility is by far the greater complicated problem. The above patents describe various approaches to the modification of the outer surface of copolymer beads. Coating the beads with poly(N-vinyl-2-pyrrolidone) or poly(vinyl alcohol) that are well known to be biocompatible materials is the first approach. These polymers are normally used as suspension stabilizers in the process of copolymerization of styrene and divinylbenzene. It is quite logical to assume that a certain portion of the stabilizer can remain adsorbed (or entangled) on the outer surface of beads thus making them rather hemocompatible. However, as we examined experimentally in direct canine tests, the washed macroporous polystyrene-type beads reveal complete absence of hemocompatibility.

More efficient should be the chemical binding of hydrophilic polymers to the bead surface and, indeed, several patents suggest covering of beads with a film of hemocompatible polymer. Hoverer, none of the patents elucidates the influence of the film on the diffusion kinetics of toxic substances to be extracted from the blood. Also, in the majority of cases the hemocompatibility of the final materials was simply declared rather than proven.

Moreover, patent authors largely disregard characteristic details of the process of grafting hydrophilic polymers on the surface of hydrophobic macroporous styrene copolymers. When such dry beads are placed in water, the latter will not fill the pores inside the polymer and even proper wetting of bead outer surface will not be secured. This casts doubts on the efficiency of modification of dry beads in aqueous media. Copolymer beads must be pre-wetted by a special treatment. On the other hand, chemical modification in an organic media (for instance, by using residual chloromethyl groups or pendent double bonds) will result in changing the chemistry of both bead surface and its macropores, which is not always beneficial for the adsorption process of substances retained due to hydrophobic interactions.

We believe that the suggestion of Davankov et al. [24] presents the most reasonable one for modifying selectively the outer surface of styrene-divinylbenzene copolymers. Here, grafting of water-soluble polar monomers to form short hemocompatible polymer chains on the surface takes place on the beads the internal volume of which is filled with water-immiscible organic solvent (diluent). This innovation permits obtaining of the final hemosorbent in a one-step preparation procedure while securing proper hydrophilisation of the outer bead surface and leaving the internal pore surface hydrophobic. The excellent hemocompatibility of materials thus obtained was proved by numerous tests on dogs and people and will be discussed in detail in the following sections.

Thus, we are drawing the conclusion that the use of commercially available macroporous styrene-divinylbenzene copolymers in the practice of hemosorption is mostly retarded by the problems of their surface modification. Besides, we believe that the trivial macroporous structure of the copolymers is far from being the optimal one for the purpose of sorption of the wide spectrum of toxic chemical and protein-type toxic compounds that are present in blood of many patients. We have every reason to state that hypercrosslinked polystyrene-type sorbents with a fundamentally different physical and porous structure present much more promising materials for preparing the most efficient non-selective hemosorbents. To elucidate this statement it seems to be reasonable to consider the basic principles of formation of macroporous and hypercrosslinked polymers as well as the fundamental difference in their structures which conditions differences in their ability to extract various toxins from blood and plasma.

3. POROUS POLYSTYRENIC ADSORBING MATERIALS

3.1. Macroporous Styrene-Divinylbenzene Copolymers

Macroporous styrene-divinylbenzene (DVB) copolymers possess two-phase (heterogeneous) structure composed of voids (pores) and dense polymeric walls. They are obtained by free radical copolymerization of styrene with rather large (more than 8 mol-%) amount of DVB in the presence of inert diluents (porogens). The latter are miscible with the comonomers, but do not dissolve the forming polymers. To prepare the final material in the form of spherical particles (beads) the suspension polymerization technique has usually been employed where the mixed solution of comonomers and an initiator of polymerization in the inert diluent is dispersed in an aqueous phase containing a suspension stabilizer. As polymerization proceeds in each separate droplet, primary nano-sized insoluble polymer particles precipitate within the initial homogeneous droplet; they aggregate, agglomerate and eventually combine to form an entire opaque solid bead. Within the bead, voids between the primary polymer nanoparticles are occupied by the porogen. The removal of the latter leaves macropores behind.

Depending on the type of the porogen one may discuss two reasons leading to the above phase separation during the polymerization procedure. The first reason consists in the thermodynamic incompatibility of growing polymeric chains and microgels with the inert diluent which proportion grows during the progressive consumption of comonomers. Aliphatic hydrocarbons and alcohols belong to the family of such polymer-incompatible diluents. The second reason for phase separation applies for the case of diluents that are thermodynamically good medium for dissolving polystyrene chains (for example, toluene or xylene). Here, at a certain threshold DVB content in the initial mixture, the damount of the good solvent present in the system may prove to be larger than the copolymer primary microparticles can accommodate. In this case the growing porogen-swollen microgel particles of styrene-DVB copolymer separate from the solution, aggregate, agglomerate, while unabsorbed excess solvent remains between the consolidating microparticles. In both cases the resulting product is composed of two segregated phases one of which is the polymer and the other is the diluent. After the removal of the latter, in the first case large pores remain between dense primary polymer nanoparticles while in the second case, in addition to the macropores, the primary particles themselves contain micropores.

In accordance with the recommendations of IUPAC (International Union of Pure and Applied Chemistry), the micropores are considered to be those having ≤20 E in diameter, mesopores have diameter between 20 E and 500 E, while the diameter of macropores exceeds 500 E. Although the conventional macroporous styrene-divinylbenzene copolymers belong in fact to the family of mesoporous materials, it is generally accepted to call them "macroporous" copolymers. (This term has appeared long before the IUPAC recommenddations and has established itself).

A large number of investigations concerning the influence of different factors on the porous structure of macroporous polymers led to the development of quite a number of neutral (non-functionalized) sorbents characterized by excellent permeability for a vide variety of organic compounds. Among them the macroporous polystyrene sorbents of Amberlite XAD series produced by Rohm & Haas Company (USA) are the most popular.

The fields of styrene-DVB copolymers' practical applications include adsorption of organics from gaseous and liquid phases, gas and liquid chromatography, preparation of ion exchange resins for large organic ions and catalysis of organic reactions, etc. At the same time, because of the high extent of crosslinking (> 8 %) of the polymeric microphase the majority of organic compounds adsorb only on the surface of macropores (specific surface area is usually smaller than 100-200 m^2/g); that is why the adsorption capacity of macroporous sorbents often proves to be insufficient for commercial applications.

3.2. Hypercrosslinked Polystyrene

In the beginning of 1970th Davankov and Tsyurupa [47] suggested a fundamentally new approach to the synthesis of polystyrene-type sorbents which combined a good permeability with a high adsorption capacity for a wide variety of organic compounds. This approach consists in the formation of a rigid, homogeneous (single-phase) highly expanded three-dimensional network. One may obtain such a kind of networks by crosslinking pre-formed polystyrene chains in solution or in highly swollen state with a large amount of rigid bridges. By using highly reactive bifunctional crosslinking agents, it proved to be possible to bind between one another almost all phenyl rings of the initial polystyrene chains, thus obtaining *homogeneous, rigid, expanded openwork structure*. Naturally, such a new material required a new name. Therefore the networks prepared in accordance with the aforementioned principle and having the degree of crosslinking higher than 40 % have got general name "hypercrosslinked" networks.

Hypercrosslinked polystyrene owes its excellent adsorption properties to the unique structure which, in its turn, is determined by the above conditions of network synthesis. Exhaustive information about hypercrosslinked polystyrene can be found in the book by the same authors "Hypercrosslinked Polymeric Networks and Adsorbing Materials" [48].

The numerous rigid bridges-struts introduced by the intensive crosslinking of relatively long polystyrene chains in solution or in a highly swollen styrene-DVB copolymer keep the polystyrene chains on a certain distance from one another both in dry and swollen material, thus assuring the formation of rigid open network structure.

Many organic compounds such as bis(chloromethyl)-derivatives of aromatic hydrocarbons, monochlorodimethyl ether or dimethoxymethane can be used as crosslinking agents that react with polystyrene in the presence of Friedel-Crafts catalysts. Figure 4.1 illustrates the principle scheme of hypercrosslinked polystyrene synthesis using, as an example, the most frequently employed two-step one-pot reaction of polystyrene with mono-chlorodimethyl ether.

Importantly, the crosslinking of polystyrene chains in solution or in highly swollen state (i.e., in a thermodynamically good solvent) is not accompanied by microphase separation but results in obtaining swollen single-phase rigid network. Indeed, before the reaction starts, all components are uniformly distributed throughout the entire volume of initial solution (or gel), and polystyrene chains are solvated by the good solvent (e.g., ethylene dichloride) both before and during the refraction. The bridging starts simultaneously in many points of contacts between polystyrene chains. In several seconds, many rigid bridges fix initial polymeric chains in space thus depriving them the possibility to approach one another and form a separate (from the solvent) polymeric phase.

In a solvated chain of atactic polystyrene two neighboring phenyl rings are twisted relative to each other by approximately 120°. If one bridge forms between two chains, the next pair of phenyls along these chains proves to be located far from each other and most likely will react with phenyls of other chains. In other words, formation of one bridge hinders the formation of neighboring bridges between phenyl groups of the same pair of chains and prevents the formation of domains with enhanced crosslinking density. The formation of uniformly crosslinked network is most probable.

All surprising properties of hypercrosslinked polystyrene manifest themselves at the degree of crosslinking no less than 40 %. In a network with 100 % crosslinking degree almost all phenyl groups are connected between one another. When crosslinking degree amounts to 200 % each phenyl ring participates twice in the bridging. To explain the special properties of so highly crosslinked network, we must imagine its structure as an openwork ensemble of mutually condensed and interpenetrating macrocycles (meshes). In a hypercrosslinked polystyrene network the smallest nearly unstressed mesh can be composed of three pairs of neighboring phenyl rings initially belonging to three different polystyrene chains and finally connected by three methylene groups (Figure 1). It is important that even this smallest mesh contains a large number of C-C bonds and in principle may change its conformation.

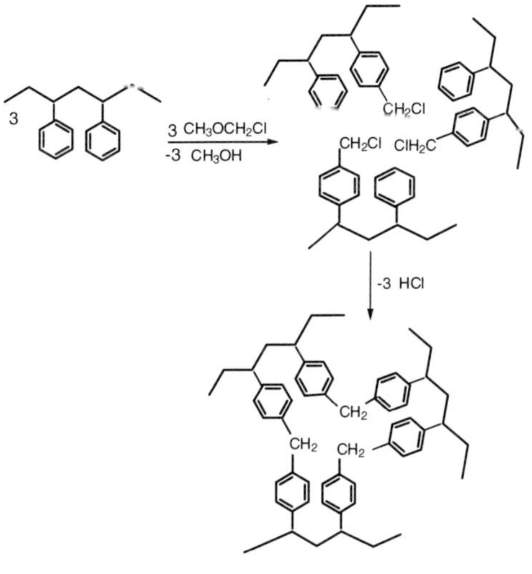

Figure 4.1. The scheme of hypercrosslinked polystyrene synthesis.

Each mesh is condensed with many neighboring meshes. Since the hypercrosslinked network has no long flexible fragments, any change in the conformation of a mesh inevitably entails changes in conformations of neighboring meshes. Concerted cooperative conformational rearrangement of a large number of meshes permits significant changes in the volume of the whole network. We can observe the network shrinkage on drying and its reversible expansion by a factor of 2 to 3 on swelling.

Two striking features distinguish the hypercrosslinked polystyrene from all other types of polystyrene structures. The first is its high porosity of a new type. Shrinkage of the network on removing the solvent from the swollen gel that results from the polymerization process, leads to a significant change in its volume. This process is combined with an enforced cooperative conformational rearrangement of meshes, which is unavoidably accompanied by appearing and rapid growth of inner stresses within each mesh and the network as a whole. Stresses are caused by the tendency of desolvated polystyrene chains to achieve dense packing, on the one hand, and the high rigidity of open network, preventing deformations, on the other hand. These inner stresses manifest themselves and stock up in the form of distorted bond lengths and valence angles. Eventually, the inner stresses equilibrate the attraction forces between desolvated network fragments and stop further shrinkage, despite the continuing solvent removal. Therefore, the final dry hypercrosslinked product differs from all other crosslinked polymeric materials in the presence of high inner stresses.

Because of inner stresses in dry hypercrosslinked polystyrene, it tends to swell and expand up to the volume in which the network was formed and which is characterized by the smallest deviations from unstressed equilibrium mesh conformations. This tendency manifests itself in the unique ability of hypercrosslinked polystyrene to swell in any gaseous and liquid media, irrespective of their thermodynamic affinity to polystyrene-precursor. Even water can occupy the interior of the hydrophobic open network causing its significant swelling.

The second distinguishing feature of hypercrosslinked polystyrene is its high porosity. The shrinkage of network on drying stops long before the achievement of chains' dense packing which is characteristic of linear polystyrene or gel-type styrene-DVB copolymers. The large free volume remaining in the dry single-phase uniformly crosslinked network can be considered as its true porosity. This is a new type of porosity. The earlier known porosity of polymeric materials resulted from phase separation during their preparation. The two-phase macroporous polymers are always opaque. In contrast, the porous hypercrosslinked polystyrene does not scatter visible light; this is a transparent material with a large number of very small (nano-sized) pores.

Porous hypercrosslinked polystyrene absorbs large amounts of inert gases at low temperature. The apparent specific inner surface area calculated on the base of nitrogen adsorption data can achieve 2000 m^2/g. However, this value reflects only the high adsorption capability of the polymer rather than its real surface area, because no real interface borders exist within the openwork single-phase hypercrosslinked network.

The size of free spaces in hypercrosslinked polystyrene is small, 1.5-3 nm (15-30 E), depending on conditions of network synthesis. These values fit somewhere between true micropores ($\leq$2 nm) and mesopores (2-50 nm) and so the hypercrosslinked polystyrene has to be considered as the first nanoporous polymeric material.

Earlier, we reported [49] that apart from polystyrene many other polymers can exhibit the specific properties of hypercrosslinked structure provided their preparation follows the basic principle of hypercrosslinked network synthesis, namely, the formation of a rigid highly solvated network. Thus, hypercross-linked polymers may be obtained by polymerization (polydivinylbenzene, styrene-DVB copolymers), polycondensation (poly-xylene, polyamides) or crosslinking of any pre-formed polymeric chains (polysulfone, polypyrrol). All of them are compatible with any liquid including water and are characterized by intrinsic microporosity. Any hypercrosslinked polymer must function as a non-specific adsorbent and exhibit high adsorption capacity.

However, for practical purposes, in particular, for hemoperfusion, one often needs materials containing not only micropores, but also large pores that facilitate the diffusion and enable adsorption of larger species as proteins. Such a kind of materials is thought to be prepared by combining of two global principles of network formation, i.e., the principle of macroporous polymer formation based on phase separation phenomenon, and that of hyper-crosslinked polymers synthesis based on intensive crosslinking of solvated chains and resulting in development of micropore system.

As will be shown later in this Chapter, the combination of the above two global principles of network formation provides polymeric materials that are most suitable for hemoperfusion. While the hypercrosslinking process resulting in the open-network microporous structure of the material determines its enhanced hemocompatibility and the high adsorption capacity towards small toxic molecules, the phase separation process during the synthesis enhances the sorption kinetics and provides sorption sites for middle-molecular-weight toxic proteins. The optimal networks must be characterized by two types of pores, "micro" and "macro". As a matter of fact, these networks also possess pores of intermediate size, "mesopores". The latter can even predominate in the total pore size distribution plot. It is these "biporous" and predominantly "mesoporous" polystyrene-type materials that we will discuss in the following.

4. HYPERCROSSLINKED POLYSTYRENE-TYPE MATERIALS AS POTENTIAL HEMOSORBENTS

Preliminary Studies

The problem whether or not biporous hypercrosslinked polystyrene and mesoporous polydivinylbenzene adsorbing materials are suitable for extracorporeal blood purification was investigated using, as the first example, the extraction of chlorinated hydrocarbons and some other xenobiotics from blood [50-52].

An acute poisoning with chlorinated hydrocarbons or toxic chemicals is one of the gravest pathologic conditions with a high hospital mortality approaching 50 %. Among the most effective methods of therapy of the severe intoxication, hemoperfusion represents the basic means that permits within a short period of time almost comprehensive elimination of toxic compounds from blood, as well as lymph and enteral medium, thus improving the projection of disease treatment.

A group of ten sorbents was chosen for comparative studies. It incurporated modified activated carbons (synthetic SKN-2M and VNIITU and SKT-6a of natural origin), carbon/mineral preparation SUMS-1, a macroporous polystyrene-DVB Polysorb, modified mesoporous styrene-DVB copolymers CCP-006 and PRI-15 as well as biporous hypercrosslinked polystyrene Styrosorb-514; the latter three sorbents belonging to the family of hypercrosslinked materials. All sorbents were from Russia. 1,2-Ethylene dichloride (EDC), methanol, trichloromethafos-3 (FOS) and phenobarbital were taken as the representatives of various toxic compounds while human serum albumin (HSA) and Methylene blue (MB) served as substitutes for bio-related sorbates. In experiments performed *in vitro*, 50 mL of citric whole donor blood containing a deadly dose of the above xenobiotics were sent through a sorbent bed of one centimeter in diameter and five mL in volume within three minutes. The concentration of each adsorbate in the filtrate was then determined by appropriate physico-chemical methods.

Table 4.1 shows the sorption efficiency of the above sorbents towards the examined xenobiotics. The general advantage of hypercrosslinked polymers is obvious, though they extract methanol and phosphorus-organic FOS still inadequately.

Sorption of Methylene blue and HSA from model aqueous solutions was examined under static conditions by incubation of 0.2 g sorbent with 50 mL of 0.15 % MB solution or 0.5 % HSA solution for one hour. It turned out, the modified activated carbons and Styrosorb-514 extract no more than 72 mg/g of HSA while one gram of CCP-006 and PRI-15 take up 216 and 237 mg of HSA, respectively. On the one hand, the high adsorption of albumin onto last two hypercrosslinked sorbents (Table 4.2) may unfavorably affect the protein status of blood. On the other hand, albumin, being a middle-size protein of 65000-67000 Da molecular weight and having about 6 nm in diameter, may serve as a convenient model for the estimation of adsorption activity of these sorbents relative to middle or higher molecular weight proteins the high plasmatic concentrations of which has always accompanied an endogenic intoxication.

Methylene blue is usually considered to be universal marker for the evaluation of hemosorbent adsorption ability towards xenobiotics with middle molecular weight. CCP-006 was found to adsorb only 72 mg/g MB whereas Styrosorb 514 is capable of adsorbing nearly twice as much amount of the dye, 125 mg/g (Table 4.3).

Table 4.1. The removal (%) of xenobiotics from a whole donor blood; the initial concentration of toxic compounds is given in brackets

Sorbent	Adsorption, %			
	1,2-EDC (100 ng/L)	**Methanol (1.3 mg/L)**	**FOS (10 mg/L)**	**Phenobarbital (100 mg/L)**
SUMC-1	84	4.7	9.7	62.4
SKN-2M	90	7.8	5.6	86.8
SKT-6a	56	13.2	10.7	>99
CCP-006	>99	22.5	39.3	>99
Styrosorb-514	>99	23.2	16.8	94.6

**Table 4.2. Adsorption capacity of the examined sorbents
for human serum albumin**

Sorbent	Adsorption capacity, mg/g
SUMS-1	19.2±2.3
AKN-2M	31.2±3.6
SKT-6a	37.4±5.3
Activated carbon OU-A (powder)	61.6±9.7
Styrosorb-514	72.2±3.0
Polyfepan	84.6±6.5
VNIITU	186.4±7.6
CCP-006	216.6±10.5
PRI-15	237.7±5.5
Polysorb	372.5±7.3

**Table 4.3. Adsorption capacity of the examined sorbents
for Methylene blue**

Adsorbent	Adsorption capacity, mg/g
Polysorb	41.7±2.9
SUMS-1	48.7±1.3
Polyfepan	48.9±9.9
SKT-6a	71.1±8.5
CCP-006	75.6±18.3
PRI-15	88.7±9.3
VNIITU	86.4±7.4
SKN-2M	89.4±5.3
Styrosorb-514	125.7±4.53
Activated carbon OU-A (powder)	255.2±9.8

The above results indicate that the hypercrosslinked polystyrene-type sorbents can effectively extract various typical toxic compounds from blood. However, it is no less important to know how a hemoperfusion process affects blood morphology and its coagulation system, for instance, on poisoning with 1,2-ethylene dichloride. The study in this direction was carried out using mongrels of 15-25 kg in weight. The animals were divided into four groups each containing eight dogs. The first group was reference one. The synthetic carbon hemosorbent with modified surface SKN-2M was employed to purify the blood of dogs belonging to the second group. The hypercrosslinked sorbents Styrosorb-514 and CCP-006 were used for the third and fourth groups of dogs, respectively. Before the cartridge was connected to blood stream, each dog received 500 units/kg heparin which was neutralized after the hemoperfusion session by the injection of coagulant, protamine sulfate. The sorbents were also treated with heparin. Three hours before hemoperfusion started, all dogs received 2000 mg/kg 1,2-EDC as oral injection. Within the following one hour, the circulating blood volume of animals in experimental groups was percolated three times through 100 mL sorption cartridges packed with sorbents under investigation. Table 4.4 reports the data characterizing both the impact of the acute poisoning with ethylene dichloride and consequences of hemoperfusion session on the morphological status of canine blood.

First of all it should be noted that hypercrosslinked surface-modified CCP-006 and Styrosorb-514 have to be considered really hemocompatible materials because within the hemoperfusion session the concentration of blood cells including platelets did not change and there was no hemolysis at all. As concerns the overall detoxification effect when judged by minimal changes of hemoglobin, platelets, erythrocytes, leukocytes and monocytes counts during hemoperfusion and 24 hours after the acute intoxication, these polymeric sorbents outperformed the efficiency of modified activated carbon hemosorbent SKN-2M. The same conclusion follows from the behavior of animals and analysis data of all hemostasis parameters.

In the reference group of animals all characteristics of blood morphology were observed to be typical for the formation and following progress in the syndrome of dissemination intravascular fibrillation which is specific for poisoning with ethylene dichloride.

Thus, all above preliminary *in vitro* and *in vivo* experiments clearly demonstrated good hemocompatibility of the mesoporous polydivinylbenzene and hypercrosslinked polystyrene sorbents and their ability to efficiently adsorb many toxic low-molecular-weight organic compounds from a whole blood. Moreover, presence of larger pores, in addition to the inherent microporosity of hypercrosslinked networks, implies their potential usefulness in removing toxic proteins.

Table 4.4. The effect of hemoperfusion on the composition of arterial canine blood after an acute poisoning with 1,2-EDC

N	Group of animals	Characteristics	3 hours after poisoning	3 hours after poisoning and 1 h hemoperfusion	24 hours after poisoning
1	No hemoper-fusion	Erythrocytes, Ч10^6/μL	4.4±0.9	5.2±0.3	5.8±1.1*
		Hemoglobin, g/L	184±16	220±13*	240±24*
		Leukocytes, Ч10^6/mL	7.4±1.2	5.1±2.6	14.0±3.2*
		Banded neutrophils, %	1.4±0.9	36.1±17.2*	26.5±4.1*
		Segmented neutrophils, %	82.0±7.1-	54.8±6.2*	58.6±2.1*
		Platelets, Ч10^6/mL	240.7±16.4	260.4±18.6	170.4±36.7*
		Lymphocytes, %	11.6±3.8	14.5±4.9	20.7±6.5*
		Monocytes, %	5.4±2.9	2.7±1.6	10.1±4.3*
		Free hemoglobin, g/L	0	16.0±6.7*	26.1±9.6*
2	Hemoper fusion on activated carbon SKN-2M	Erythrocytes, Ч10^6/μL	5.2±0.5	4.5±0.4	4.7±0.7
		Hemoglobin, g/L	185±11	180±16	187±26
		Leukocytes, Ч10^6/mL	11.2±1.7	14.2±0.9	13.9±4.1
		Banded neutrophils, %	5.5±2.6	5.0±2.6	14.0±4.3*
		Segmented neutrophils, %	61.0±5.7	68.5±3.6	71.0±18.0
		Platelets, Ч10^6/mL	171.5±18.8	107.2±10,8*	98.2±8.3*
		Lymphocytes, %	12.5±5.4	14.5±7.5	5.0±2.7*
		Monocytes, %	3.2±0.7	3.0±0.4	5.1±1.1*
		Free hemoglobin, g/L	0	14.7±6.4*	13.5±6.7*
3	Hemoper fusion on Styrosorb-514	Erythrocytes, Ч10^6/μL	5.2±0.2	5.4±0.9	5.6±1.1
		Hemoglobin, g/L	180±17	182±19	170±28
		Leukocytes, Ч10^6/mL	8.0±1.1	12.6±2.0*	11.4±0.9*
		Banded neutrophils, %	5.0±0.8	6.2±1.6	11.0±0.8*
		Segmented neutrophils, %	67.6±4.0	77.8±3.6	58.3±4.5
		Platelets, Ч10^6/mL	270.8±14.0	281.6±15.2	210.4±36.1*
		Lymphocytes, %	8.0±3.1	12.4±6.8	12.4±2.1
		Monocytes, %	2.8±1.4	12.8±8.6*	10.4±6.2*
		Free hemoglobin, g/L	0	0	7.0±1.4*
4	Hemoper fusion on CCP-006	Erythrocytes, Ч10^6/μL	4.6±1.1	3.9±0.8	4.5±0.7
		Hemoglobin, g/L	148.6±23.7	149.6±17.4	142.6±19.6
		Leukocytes, Ч10^6/mL	12.7±6.3	18.4±4.8	20.4±4.7
		Banded neutrophils, %	6.0±0.7	5.2±0.9	9.4±1.7*
		Segmented neutrophils, %	68.7±8.4	70.6±3.7	74.2±6.9
		Platelets, Ч10^6/mL	200.6±24.9	200.7±31.7	170.1±24.6
		Lymphocytes, %	17.2±4.2	19.4±3.0	10.2±3.6*
		Monocytes, %	7.0±1.1	6.1±0.9	6.2±2.3
		Free hemoglobin, g/L	0	0	2,5±0,2

* statistical significance p<0,05.

5. REMOVAL OF TOXINS FROM THE BLOOD OF PATIENTS WITH KIDNEY FAILURE

5.1. Hypercrosslinked Styrene-Divinylbenzene Copolymers for the Removal of B_2-Microglobulin

For the removal of middle-size toxic proteins, most desirable should be hemocompatible hydrophobic polymeric sorbents with an enhanced proportion of mesopores, in the range from 4 to 10 nm. The majority of hypercrosslinked adsorbing resins obtained by bridging linear polystyrene chains in solution or crosslinking swollen styrene-divinylbenzene copolymers represent transparent materials with nanopores of 1.5-3.0 nm in diameter.

Copolymerization of divinylbenzene was thought to offer the opportunity of preparing beaded adsorbing materials with the desired size of pores. It has been well documented that the phase separation during the formation of a rigid polymeric network in the course of copolymerization of monomers, in particular, styrene and divinylbenzene, in the presence of a diluent that is miscible with monomers but precipitates the formed polymer, results in obtaining a macroporous material. On the contrary, largely microporous structures are formed if the copolymerization proceeds in the presence of a diluent which is compatible with both the comonomers and the resulting polymer. No phase separation takes place if the amount of such diluent is relatively small. When the proportion of the latter exceeds the swelling ability of the final rigid network the excess solvent forms a separate phase, thus introducing additional larger pores.

When taking into account the above reasons for phase separation, it is logical to suppose that required mesoporous networks could form if the diluent represents an organic medium with a thermodynamic quality situated between good solvents and precipitants for the polymer. Indeed, preparation of hypercrosslinked networks by crosslinking linear polystyrene chains dissolved in cyclohexane, a rather poor solvent for polystyrene even at the temperature of synthesis, 60 °C, resulted in obtaining basically mesoporous materials having an exceptionally high adsorption capacity, also with respect to β_2-microglobulin. Unfortunately, we failed, thus far, to prepare these materials in a beaded form of sufficient mechanical strength.

In accordance with the above principles, polymerization of divinylbenzene in the presence of a diluent having an intermediate thermodynamic quality has been intensively studied and, indeed, resulted in obtaining mesoporous materials. In order to develop a rigid network of the desired porosity, DVB (usually more than 30 % in its mixture with styrenic comonomers) must be copolymerized in the presence of a sufficient amount of a diluent (usually 100 % or more of the volume of the comonomers). Of crucial importance is the nature and composition of the diluent. Beside cyclohexane, mixtures of a thermodynamically good solvent (ethylene dichloride, toluene, xylene, etc.) with precipitating media (hexane, octane, isooctane, higher aliphatic alcohols, etc.), taken in an appropriate proportion, can be applied. Phase separation during the free radical copolymerization in such a mixture should take place when the major part of the comonomers has converted into polymer.

If the network structure is rigid enough to prevent the collapse of the bead on removing the diluent after the synthesis, the total volume of pores and voids in the final polymer approaches the volume of the porogen in the mixture under polymerization. In our experiments, a series of copolymers was obtained with the total porosity varying between 1.0 and 1.7 cm^3/g and an apparent specific surface area of 550 to 800 m^2/g. Pore size distribution calculated from adsorption isotherms for nitrogen at low temperature was found to be sensitive to the composition of the initial mixture under polymerization as well as the polymerization protocol. Broad pore size distribution with a diffuse maximum located between 15 and 25 nm is typical for the polymers obtained. A sufficiently large portion of pores with smaller diameters revealed itself in the high adsorption capacity towards smaller toxic molecules, which is generally characteristic of hypercrosslinked polystyrene materials. The typical property of hypercrosslinked networks, namely the swelling in any liquid media, was also strongly expressed. The volume of dried polymers increased by a factor of at least 1.3 when the interior of beads was filled with water and 1.5 when they were wetted with methanol (non-solvents for polystyrene), with a further smaller volume increase on substituting methanol for a good solvent, such as toluene. Contrary to this, typical macroporous styrene-DVB copolymers are known to maintain their volume constant, both in a dry or wetted state.

The mechanical strength of the mesoporous polymers was found to be good. Each bead of 0.4 mm in diameter could tolerate a load as high as 300 to 450 g before destruction. Strength is an important parameter, since crushed particles and fines released from an adsorbent bed could embolize into the patient's circulation. The optimal bead size of the polymeric adsorbent was found to be 0.3-0.8 mm, which prevented high back pressures at moderate to high flow rates of viscous liquids, such as whole blood and plasma, through a 200-300 mL cartridge packed with the polymer.

The important property of the above mesoporous hypercrosslinked polystyrene-polydivinylbenzene-type materials is their high adsorption capacity towards small proteins and lower affinity to large protein molecules, probably due to size exclusion effects. Cytochrome C, which has a molecular weight of 13 kDa, was used as a substitute for β_2-microglobulin (11.8 kDa) in the adsorption experiments. From a twenty-fold volume of a very dilute solution of Cytochrome C in a neutral phosphate buffer, the polymer easily removed 70-98 % of the protein. This corresponds to an adsorption capacity of 11 to 14 mg of protein per 1 mL of wet beads, or approximately 30 mg per 1 g of dry polymer. In contrast to Cytochrome C, adsorption of larger albumin molecules from a 20-fold volume of relatively concentrated solutions (35 mg/mL) was found to be moderate, about 5 to 7 % of the initial amount [53].

Materials which were rated good in screening tests with Cytochrome C and albumin, removed 95 % of $\beta_2 M$ and less than 5 % of albumin and other essential proteins during *in vitro* tests with blood or plasma of end-stage renal dialysis patients (Figure 4.2).

A relatively high apparent selectivity of $\beta_2 M$ removal compared to that of albumin appears to be caused by the difference in their size and a larger hydrophilicity of the latter protein. Indeed, the majority of pores in the mesoporous adsorbent are accessible to relatively small β_2-microglobulin molecules (MW 11.8 kDa, 3.35 nm in diameter) while the larger molecules of albumin (MW 66 kDa, 6.0 nm in diameter) can adsorb only in large pores. Because of the specificity of the problem under discussion, the most important here is the percent of proteins' initial concentrations reduction, rather than the absolute amounts of these proteins adsorbed. The loss of a few grams of albumin per treatment session can be easily tolerated by the patient, provided that most of β_2-M is eliminated.

With the initial concentrations of albumin and $\beta_2 M$ differing by nearly three orders of magnitude (circa 40 g/L and 60 mg/L, respectively), the apparent size selectivity of any adsorption process must be principally higher than that of dialysis. Indeed, in the course of a sorption process, the sorption sites that are attainable to albumin or other major plasma components will soon be saturated, while sorption sites for $\beta_2 M$ remain far from saturation till the very end of the hemoperfusion session. Therefore, the ratio of $\beta_2 M$/albumin adsorbed will steadily improve with the continuation of the procedure. In contrast, the loss of major protein components in a dialysis process will continue at a rather constant rate throughout the entire procedure, whereas the removal of $\beta_2 M$ will slow down with its concentration decreasing.

In other words, with the longer continuation of the procedure, adsorption will predominantly remove the minor component of a mixture, whereas long-term dialysis will predominantly affect the major component. This is not surprising, since dialysis is a steady dynamic process that is entirely governed by the concentration gradients of the components across the membrane (and kinetics of their through-pore diffusion), whereas the adsorption process for the major component stops on approaching the thermodynamic equilibrium for that component.

In closing this section, we should refer to the recently appeared publication of our followers from Great Britain [54], in which the synthesis of mesoporous poly-DVB and the characterization of its porous structure were reported. The polymer readily adsorbs another surrogate for B_2M, Lyzocyme of hen egg white with molecular weight of 14 kDa and size of about 4 nm, but exhibits a pretty low affinity to human serum albumin. At present, however, it is hard to tell something about any prospect of a real application of this sorbent because no information is available on its hemocompatibility.

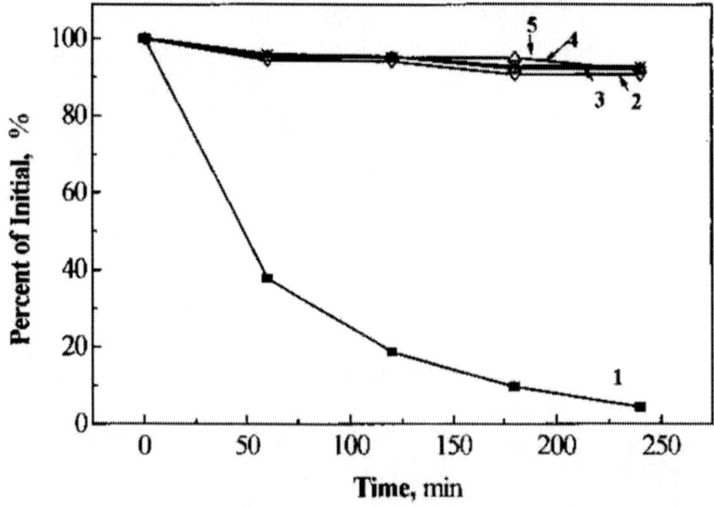

Figure 4.2. Selectivity of protein sorption on the hypercrosslinked mesoporous DVB-polymer in dynamic *in vitro* experiment with plasma. Experimental conditions: the polymer to plasma ratio is 1:20 (v/v). 37 °C, initial concentrations of proteins are as follows: (1) B_2-microglobulin – 6.35 mg/dL, (2) albumin – 3.15 g/dL, (3) prealbumin - 30 mg/dL, (4) transferin – 317 mg/dL, (5) total protein – 6.2 g/dL [53].

5.2. Hemocompatibility of Hypercrosslinked Copolymers

In vitro and in vivo studies

During blood contact with any foreign material, several components in the blood are activated through a variety of enzymatic and cellular processes. The immune system of patients with renal failure, which are forced to spend up to 15 hours weekly on hemodialysis, appears to be in a constantly activated, inflammatory state. Some doctors have suggested that the high incidence of infection and septicemia in these patients is due, in part, to the activated immune system's inability to adequately respond to microbial pathogens. Therefore, the search for the most biocompatible materials for hemodialysis and hemoperfusion is of great importance for this type of patients.

Previous experience with commercially available polystyrene-type adsorbent materials (Amberlite XAD-4) in clinical hemoperfusion was characterized by significant hemoincompatible responses, such as complement activation and sharp drop of white blood cell and platelet counts (neutropenia and thrombocytopenia). This was believed to be due to the hydrophobic nature of polystyrene surface. Similar problems were also noted with activated carbon adsorbents. The biocompatibility of the both materials needed to be improved by applying more hydrophilic polymers as surface coatings with dip or spray methods [8]. The major drawback of these surface coatings was that they tended to sharply reduce the efficiency of adsorption.

It has been noted rather early that hypercrosslinked polystyrene does not adsorb proteins to the same extent as do conventional polystyrene or macroporous polystyrene [55]. Most probably, the openwork hypercrosslinked material does not expose a dense hydrophobic surface for the proteins to adsorb. The same is true for the marked inertness of both the hypercrosslinked mesoporous polydivinylbenzene materials (prepared as mentioned above) and the hypercrosslinked sorbent Styrosorb-514 toward whole blood cells. Blood (50 mL) spiked with citric acid freely flows through a 5 mL column filled with beads of the above sorbents. Contrary to this, many other coated carbon-type and polymeric hemosorbents tested under identical conditions, caused the blood coagulation and column clotting [50]. Indeed, the new mesoporous polydivinylbenzene sorbent, without any additional modification of the surface, was found to be sufficiently hemocompatible and did not cause any early coagulation effect in a standard plasma recalcification test.

Still, further enhancement of the hemocompatibility of the polymer that is intended for a prolonged treatment of end-stage renal disease patients was thought to be important. Therefore, the outer surface of polymer beads as well as that of larger pores was subjected to chemical modification. It has been previously recognized that the consumption of vinyl groups of divinylbenzene in its polymers and copolymers is never complete. Up to 30 % of DVB involved in polymerization fails to function as a divinyl crosslinking agent and retains one of its vinyl groups intact. It is logical to assume that the pendant vinyl groups of DVB concentrate on the polymer surface, because there, they failed to find a partner for the reaction during the polymerization process. It is convenient to use these surface exposed vinyl groups to make the surface more hydrophilic and hemocompatible. As was mentioned above, we developed several simple surface modification procedures [27-30] among which the grafting of short flexible hydrophilic polymer chains by radical graft-polymerization of N-vinylpyrrolidone seems to be the most suitable. It is difficult to follow and quantitate such chemical transformations by conventional analytical techniques, unless large amounts of functional polymers are grafted onto the surface. Nevertheless, the success of the hydrophilization is always evident from the behavior of the dry polymer with respect to water [24]. Whereas the untreated dry porous material is hydrophobic and remains floated on the surface of water plus small amount of dioxane or ethanol, the modified material is hydrophilic and easily sinks in the solution. These methods of minor surface modification provide the required hemocompatibility without compromising the adsorption kinetics of the material toward small protein molecules.

The modified polymer beads passed [56] all of the standard battery of biocompatibility tests required by the International Organization for Standardization guidelines (ISO 10993). The tests included *in vitro* coagulation tests (plasma recalcification time), hemolysis study (extraction method), cytotoxicity study using the ISO elution method, etc. In *in vivo* experiments, extracts of the polymer beads did not elicit pyrogenic irritation or sensitization reactions in laboratory animals (acute systematic toxicity study in the mouse, acute intracutaneous reactivity study in the rabbit, rabbit pyrogen study).

As further evidence of the modified polymer's excellent hemo-compatibility, *in vivo* trials incorporating the polymer into a hemoperfusion device were conducted at the University of California at Davis. A polycarbonate cartridge containing 100 ml of the polymer was steam autoclaved at 120 °C for 45 minutes and flushed with one liter of sterile saline prior to use. Several times two healthy dogs underwent 5 hours of hemoperfusion at a flow rate of 200 mL/min. No adverse effects such as fever or hypotension were noted. Temperature, blood pressure, mixed venous oxygen saturation, and hematocrit were continuously monitored during the procedure and all remained unchanged throughout the procedure.

Neutropenia and thrombocytopenia are commonly observed phenomena during extracorporeal blood circulation and are considered to be the most sensitive markers of hemocompatibility. The graphs of white blood cell and platelet counts in the above canine experiments showed a characteristic reduction (by 13 and 27 %, respectively) at 15-30 minutes. To generate data for comparison, the same dogs were also subjected to 5 hours of hemodialysis under identical conditions with a modified cellulose dialyzer. In both the dialyzer and hemoperfusion experiments, white blood cell counts quickly return to normal and remain unchanged till the end of the procedure. Interestingly, platelet counts also returned to normal in the hemoperfusion group but remained low in the dialyzer group. This would suggest superior hemocompatibility of the surface modified mesoporous polydivinylbenzene adsorbent beads. With this respect it is important to note that, contrary to canine blood, no changes occurred in the platelet and leukocyte counts when human volunteer blood passed over the resin *ex vivo* [57] or *in vivo* in man during clinical hemoperfusion, as will be shown below.

5.3. Clinical Trials with Hypercrosslinked Polydivinylbenzene BetaSorb™ Polymer

Excellent sorption capacity of the hypercrosslinked mesoporous polydivinylbenzene with respect to selective removal of β_2-microglobulin from its mixtures with albumin and other serum proteins, combined with superior hemocompatibility of the bead surface modified with poly(N-vinyl)pyrrolidone, justified the manufacturing of an experimental batch of the material for initial clinical studies. The polymer was named BetaSorb™ (RenalTech International, USA) and was used in 300 mL cylindrical polysulfone devices that were steam sterilized and filled with normal saline containing 1,000 IU heparin. The device was placed in line with the dialysis circuit, upstream of the dialyzer, in order not to affect the pressure drop across the dialyzer membrane. The blood flow was maintained at the customary value of 400 mL/min, again the optimal flow rate for the dialyzer. The complete setup of the combined hemoperfusion-hemodialysis treatment [58] is displayed in Figure 4.3.

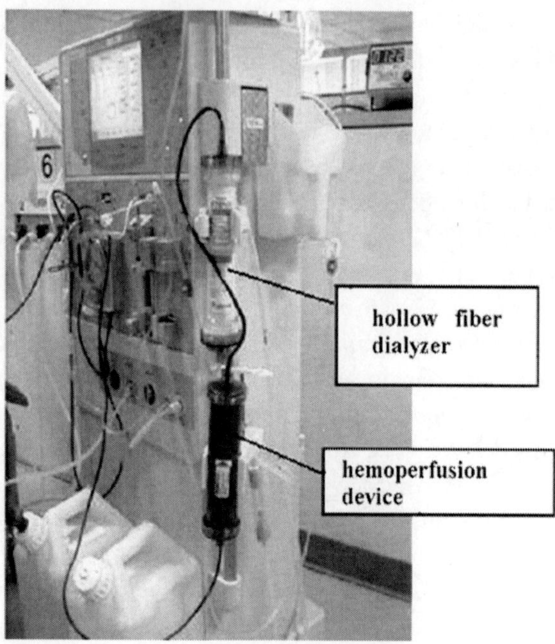

Figure 4.3. Operational unit for blood purification.

The first experiments with two end-stage renal disease, ESRD, patients at a hospital in Vicenza (Italy) clearly demonstrated full safety and efficiency of the BetaSorb^{TM} device [58]. During each of the three hour treatments platelet and leukocyte counts remained stable, as did serum albumin concentrations. In fact, these figures even increased during the session because of the removal of excess water from the circulation through dialysis membranes. On the contrary, β_2-microglobulin levels dropped by 70 and 80 % from their initial levels. Interestingly, these levels slightly rebound in 30 minutes after the hemoperfusion process. This finding indicates that an active exchange of small protein molecules exists between different compartments of physiological liquids in the organism. Therefore, it is principally possible to remove in one treatment session more of the toxin than initially circulated with blood. It also encourages the continual use of hemoperfusion in regular dialysis procedures with the hope of prevention or even reversal of dialysis related amyloidosis. Indeed, after the treatment period of three and six weeks (the time allotted for the two patients), where on the average 140 mg of $\beta_2 M$ were removed per session, a 30 % sustained reduction of the pre-dialysis $\beta_2 M$ levels were registered in 1 patient for a period of three to weeks [59]. In addition to β_2-

microglobulin, the adsorptive resin was also found to remove during the hemoperfusion session other middle molecular weight toxins, such as TNF-α (17.2 kDa) and IL-1β (17 kDa) [58], leptin (16 kDa), angiogenin (homologues to degranulation inhibitory protein I Dip1, 14.4 kDa) and several cytokines [59]. In fact, nearly 70 'classical' and 'new' uremic toxins have been found to accumulate in blood of ESRD patients [60]. Among them recent studies have identified a number of proteins, including those larger in size than β_2M, which are believed to relate to malnutrition of renal failure patients, affect their immune system or cause cardiovascular problems. Many of the toxic proteins result from the fact that hemodialysis patients are constantly exposed to a microinflammatory environment. Indeed, exposure to bacterial contaminants from dialysis water system, poorly biocompatible dialyzer membranes and tubings, and bacterial infections induce the release of pro-inflammatory cytokines, which generate chronic inflammatory state and then an acute phase reaction. Only the low molecular weight toxins are being removed during regular dialysis, but not the 'middle molecular weight' toxins with MW > 1500 Da. Adsorption of the latter by the BetaSorb^{TM} device may sufficiently increase the therapeutic effect of a combined hemoperfusion/hemodialysis treatment [60-62].

Much more extended clinical studies with BetaSorb^{TM} device were performed in the USA. Averaged data for 100 patients are as follows:

Initial concentration of β_2-microglobulin, mg/L	34 ±18.5
Total reduction of β_2M,%	70.6±10.3
Final concentration of β_2M after 30 min rebound, mg/L	14
Total removal of β_2M per session, mg	402±142

No complications related to the combined hemoperfusion/hemodialysis sessions were registered. The treatment was well received by the patients. These results speak for themselves. They prove both high safety and efficiency of the hemoperfusion procedures on hypercrosslinked polydivinylbenzene.

Long-term consequences of adding the adsorption device to the conventional hemodialysis system in treating renal patients still remain to be evaluated. For many decades, hemodialysis remains the most effective method of supporting patients with renal failure. In the United States alone in year 2000, over 15 billion dollars was spent on patients with chronic kidney failure. The cost of the dialysis treatment represents only 30 % of these expenditures. The remainder pays for the morbidity related to chronic kidney failure, problems such as dialysis-related amyloidosis, infections, nerve dysfunction, and malnutrition. Most probably, providing modern expensive hemodialysis machines with additional disposable cost-efficient hemoperfusion cartridges could contribute much to reducing this remaining 70 % portion of the costs and improving the quality of living with kidney failure [62, 63].

6. HYPERCROSSLINKED POLYMERS FOR THE REMOVAL OF TOXINS FROM BLOOD OF PATIENTS WITH SEPSIS

6.1. Hypercrosslinked Polydivinylbenzene CytoSorb™ for Treatment of Sepsis

Though the cost of treating sepsis patients in the USA was $14.6 billion in 2008, according to the Centers for Disease Control and Prevention, it remains the leading cause for mortality in intensive care units. Sepsis is a complex sequence of interrelated effects caused by the overproduction of multiple mediators and their unrestrained biological activity. The disease has usually been accompanied by uncontrolled rise in patient blood of multiple toxic proteins, cytokines, the known representatives of which are numerous interleukins (IL). The reduction of cytokines level in blood by hemoperfusion through a hypercrosslinked polystyrene-type adsorbent was found to be a powerful tool to improve the survival of patients in sepsis [64-67].

CytoSorb™ [68] is one of the family of hypercrosslinked mesoporous polydivinylbenzenes specially designed to adsorb cytokines with molecular weight of 10 to 50 kDa. It is a highly porous beaded material having pores ranging from 2 to 70 nm in diameter and specific surface area of 500-700 m^2/g. Its excellent hemocompatibility was confirmed by numerous *in vitro* and *in vivo* experiments.

Table 4.5 documents the superb adsorption ability of CytoSorb™ towards cytokines. In these experiments 8 ml of horse serum spiked with 1000-5000 pg/mL of individual cytokines were recirculated through 1 mL CytoSorb™ cartridge for 4 hours with a flow rate of about 1 mL/min [68].

One can easily note the size differentiation effect on sorption of cytokines. While smaller cytokines are completely removed from filtrated plasma, 45 % of the largest toxic protein tested, TNF-б trimer, having the molecular weight (51 kDa) close to that of albumin (66 kDa), still remains in the polymer-equilibrated plasma. Nevertheless, the result must be rated as optimum, since further increase in pore diameters of the sorbent would cause an undesirable loss of albumin.

CtytoSorb™ was evaluated in the CytoSorbents' (USA) European Sepsis Trial – a randomized, controlled, multi-center study in Germany in 43 patients with septic shock and respiratory failure (predominantly acute respiratory distress syndrome). CytoSorb™ plus standard of care (SOC) therapy achieved the primary endpoint of the trial, demonstrating the statistically significant 30-50 % reduction of many key cytokines compared to standard of care therapy alone. Indeed, as an example, Table 4.6 shows the results of one series of experiments. Patients with septic shock and respiratory failure were treated with a standard CytoSorb™ device for six hours a day for seven consecutive days (each day with a new device) at flow rates of 200-300 mL/min. While in patients treated with the sorbent under study the percent reduction of plasma cytokine levels taken from a whole blood across the 4-day and 7-day periods amounts to 30-70 % and 10-70 %, respectively, in a control group of patients which received standard of care therapy the concentration of cytokines, on the contrary, rises on average by 40-60 %.

Table 4.5. The removal of a broad spectrum of cytokines by hemoperfusion on CytoSorb™

Cytokines	Molecular weight, kDa	Percent removal
IL-8	8	100
IL-1a	17	100
IL-16	17	100
IL-10	18	85
IL-6	26	87
HMGB1	30	80
TNF6 trimer	51	55

Table 4.6. Percent reduction of cytokine levels by CytoSorb™ plus standard of care therapy *versus* standard of care therapy alone [68]

Cytokines	CytoSorb™ + SOC		SOC alone	
	4th day	7th day	4th day	9th day
IL-6	- 45	- 40	+ 50	+ 125
IL-8	- 30	+ 10	+ 50	+ 25
IL-1a	- 70	- 70	+ 50	0
NCP-1	- 40	- 40	+ 120	+ 20

"-" means decrease in cytokine level, "+" means increase in cytokine levels.

The CytoSorb™ treatment of patients with highly elevated level of IL-6 ($\geq$ 1,000 pg/mL) or IL-1a ($\geq$ 6,000 pg/mL) which are known to be independent predictors of mortality in sepsis, resulted in statistically significant reduction in 28-day all-cause mortality: 0 % *versus* 63 % in control group of patients treated conventionally (p=0.03, n=14) and a trend to benefit in 60-day mortality, namely, 17 % *vs* 63 % control (p=0.14, n=14).

CytoSorb™ therapy is safe and well-tolerated. The sorbent does not impact delicately balanced blood chemistries. It is applicable for patients with or without renal failure. It has been used in more than 650 human treatments without serious device-related adverse effects. At present, CytoSorb™ represents the first-class hypercrosslinked adsorbing material specifically approved as an extracorporeal cytokine filter in the European Union [68].

CytoSorbents Corporation (USA) that optimized the hypercrosslinked sorbent CytoSorb™ for detoxification of blood of patients with sepsis, further suggests a new and witty way of using a hypercrosslinked hemocompatible polydivinylbenzene polymer for general blood purification. The corporation named this way HemoDefend technology platform [68]. The fact is that annually US hospitals require 15 million packed red blood cell (pRBC) transfusions, an estimated 50 million pRBC transfusions worldwide. Transfusion of platelets, plasma, cryoprecipitate and other blood products double this number. Trauma, surgery, critical care illnesses, cancer, military usage, and inherited blood disorders are just some of the drivers of transfused blood products.

However, transfusion is not so simple procedure. There is a low but still tangible (1-4 %) risk of non-hemolytic febrile and allergic transfusion reactions, undefined risks of allo-immunization, risk of atypical infection, such as prions, the infectious agent responsible for Creutzfeldt-Jakob, or "mad-cow" disease, and risk of potentially fatal transfusion reactions including transfusion related acute lung injury, 1 in 2,000 to 5,000 transfusions, anaphylaxis (1 in 20,000-50,000), angioedema, and hemolysis. Transfusion risk increases in patients receiving multiple pRBC units (e.g. trauma, surgery) and in "primed" susceptible patients (e.g. critical care and high risk surgery).

Donated blood can contain foreign antigens, antibodies, medications, infectious materials (e.g. prions, viruses) and other substances that can cause serious consequences. During blood storage, pRBC units also accumulate free hemoglobin due to hemolysis, and undergo in situ generation of bioactive lipids (e.g. lysophosphatidylcholine), cytokines, and other inflammatory mediators that can trigger transfusion reactions depending on the patient's condition. HemoDefend is a powerful blood purification technology platform that removes antibodies, free hemoglobin, cytokines, toxins, drugs, bioactive lipids, and other inflammatory mediators thereby reducing nuisance transfusion reactions, maintaining the quality and safety of fresh blood and potentially extending the useful life of blood. HemoDefend may be used in two configurations, as in-line filter between the blood bag and the patient and as "Beads in Blood". In the latter configuration, the beads are placed directly into a blood storage bag during bag manufacturing. They immediately begin to remove contaminants from the blood and continue functioning throughout the entire blood storage period.

6.2. Hypercrosslinked Polystyrene Sorbents Styrosorb Designed for Treatment of Sepsis

In vitro and in vivo tests

Hypercrosslinked polystyrene adsorbing materials [48] of Styrosorb series (developed by authors of present Chapter in the early 1970th) are known to be neutral highly porous polymers having a variable spectrum of pores between 0.2 nm and 60 nm in diameter and high apparent specific surface area of around 1000 m^2/g. Contrary to conventional macroporous copolymers in the structure of which there exists a real boundary between a densely packed polymeric phase of rigid pore walls and space filled with air or liquid, in the single-phase hypercrosslinked polystyrenes such a boundary does not exist. Here, virtually all polystyrene chains are separated from one another by numerous rigid struts and are therefore fully exposed to a surrounding medium. The openwork structure of hypercrosslinked polystyrenes provides an easy access of low and middle molecular weight compounds to plural adsorption sites. Materials of this kind pose an extremely strong uncompensated force field and are capable of retaining a wide variety of polar and non-polar organic compounds. For these reasons the adsorption capacity of hypercrosslinked polystyrenes exceeds many times that of conventional macroporous styrene-divinylbenzene adsorbing resins. Thereupon, it was of great importance to estimate the suitability of hypercrosslinked polystyrene sorbents Styrosorb for extracorporeal blood purification.

Four specially designed samples of hypercrosslinked polystyrenes with an enhanced proportion of mesopores and partially modified surface were in comparative study, Styrosorb 414, Styrosorb 514, Styrosorb 516 and Styrosorb 514M. The first three resins are beaded materials differing in surface chemistry, pore size and pore size distribution, the latter sorbent is a composite material containing nano-particles of ferric oxides (6.7±3.8 nm, 8.7-8.9 % Fe) in the hypercrosslinked polystyrene matrix. For comparison reasons properties of commercial granulated activated carbon hemosorbent Adsorba 300C (Sweden) were also examined.

All sorbents under comparison have similar particle size (smaller than 1 mm) but different shapes. As seen from Figure 4.4, polymeric materials present regular spheres with a rather narrow particle size distribution around 0.6-0.7 mm in diameter, colored yellow to brown (for Styrosorb 514M). Surfaces of the beads and their cleavages are smooth and do not reveal any pores larger than 50 nm. Granules of activated carbon look like tiny cylinders of 2x0.8 mm with their modified surface being obviously denser than their interior where pores of several micron dominate the structure.

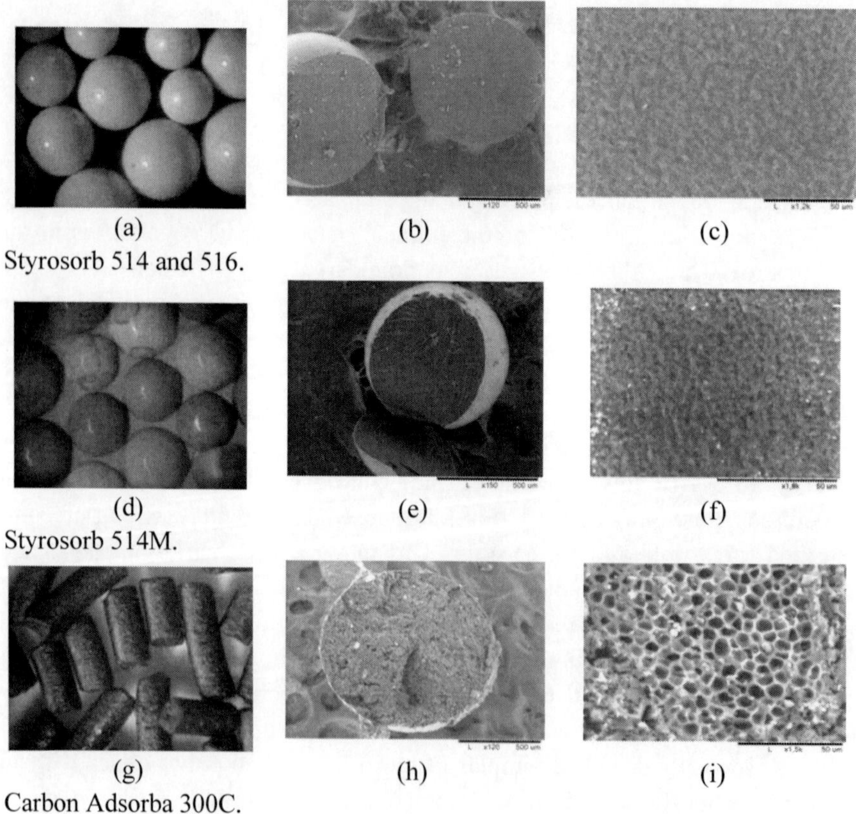

(a)   (b)   (c)

Styrosorb 514 and 516.

(d)   (e)   (f)

Styrosorb 514M.

(g)   (h)   (i)

Carbon Adsorba 300C.

Figure 4.4. Optical and scanning electron micrographs of hemosorbents under comparison.

More important is that all Styrosorb beads are rigid, mechanically and chemically stable, produce no leachables or particulates; the material is free of fines. On the contrary, activated carbons, though surface modified, are mechanically weak and generate fine particles on attrition. Carbon dust and fines on the surface of large particles is clearly seen in micrographs of Adsorba 300C [69]. (It could be mentioned here that in this respect, activated carbons obtained by pyrolysis of beaded hypercrosslinked polystyrene sulfonated resin MN500HS or conventional macroporous sulfonated ion exchange resin CT275, have much better mechanical strength, 0.7-1.2 kg per bead [70]. They were reported to have specific surface area between 700 and 900 m^2/g, well-developed mesoporosity and ability to adsorb cytokine IL-1в. However, nothing was mentioned about their hemocompatibility).

Already very first sorption experiments under static equilibration conditions have demonstrated encouraging results for the Styrosorb series of materials. As Table 4.7 demonstrates [71], from a saline solution Styrosorb 414, Styrosorb 514 and Styrosorb 516 take up well human recombinant cytokines, with the exception of interleukin IL-6 having the highest molecular weight. Most probably, the low adsorption capacity in this case is caused by insufficient accessibility of beads interior for that large protein macro-molecule.

Even better elimination effects for cytokines were observed in dynamic experiments where cytokine-spiked solutions in saline and plasma were sent through small cartridges packed with sorbents under comparison.

Beside cytokines, all hypercrosslinked sorbents actively absorb endotoxin lipopolysaccharide (LPS) *E.coli*. Under the same conditions from the solution in saline with the initial LPS concentration of 6,25±1,42 U/mL Styrosorbs 514, 414 and 516 extract 77 %, 78 % and 54 % endotoxin, respectively. As a whole, Styrosorb 514 has shown the best results; activated carbon Adsorba 300C and, in particular, Styrosorb 414 were less efficient for several types of cytokines [71]. For these reasons in the following experiments we showed preference to Styrosorb 514.

Surprising and extremely important proved to be the ability of hypercrosslinked polystyrene sorbents Styrosorb to suppress the growth of gram-positive bacteria. In *in vitro* experiment, 450 mL blood of healthy donors were spiked with gram-positive (*S. aureus*) or gram-negative (*K. pneum. pneumoniae*) microorganisms and allowed to circulate five times through 10 mL columns packed with Styrosorbs. Then, the blood aliquot was sowed on a nutrient medium and in 24 hours the number of colonies was calculated. Figure 4.5 shows 88 % decrease in the number of colonies *S. aureus* after hemoperfusion through Styrosorb 414. The contact of blood with Styrosorb 514 and Styrosorb 516 also led to sharp decrease in the number of grown colonies, by 63 % and 51 % respectively. At the same time the growth of gram-negative *K. pneum. pneumoniae* was suppressed by far the smaller extent. The largest effect, 21 %, was achieved for Styrosorb 414 while Styrosorbs 514 and 516 reduced the bacteria growth only by 2 % and 10 %, respectively [72].

Table 4.7. The concentration of cytokines (pg/mL) in physiological solutions after their incubation with the sorbents Styrosorb

Cytokines		Sorbents			Initial concentration
Type	Molecular weight, kDa	Styrosorb 516	Styrosorb 414	Styrosorb 514	
IL-8	8	232±15,1	718±15,2	196±3,5	724±22,0
IL-4	15	40±13,3	85±6,4	70±6,5	497±8,3
TNFб	17.4	265±28,7	513±13,0	86±6,4	778±25,2
IL-1в	17	88±22,3	120±22,0	112±7,5	799±26,5
IL-10	18.6	203±13,6	273±17,9	340±13.6	701±20,6
TNFв	18.6	189±20,3	516±14,3	120±1,3	860±24,1
IL-6	20.8	610±18,1	694±21,3	610±17,5	701±19,6

Experimental conditions: 35 mg sorbent, 5 mL saline, spiked with individual cytokines, incubation in shaker for 1 hour at ambient temperature. Here and thereafter the statistical significance p<0.05.

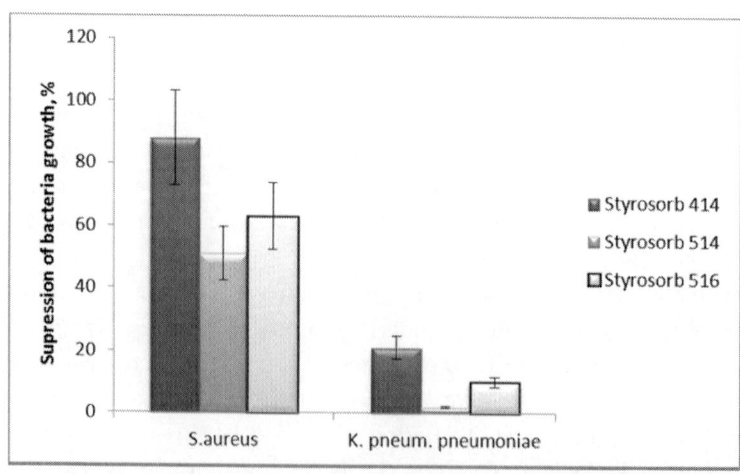

Figure 4.5. Percent of suppression of microorganism's growth after blood contacting Styrosorb polymers.

Currently, the real reason for this pretty unusual effect is not yet clear. In any case, it is hard to assume that the decrease in bacteria growth is caused by the binding of these large microorganisms in mesopores of the above hypercrosslinked sorbents or adsorption of cells on the (negligible) outer surface of sorbent beads. In fact, the ability of bacteria to form colonies is well known to be determined by proteins associated with cell surface. Some of gram-positive bacterial surface proteins determine the adhesive properties of the cells and, in particular, their virulence. Many gram-positive bacteria, such as *B. subtilis* or *L. acidophilus*, have a surface layer of proteins (40 to 60 kDa molecular weight) characterized by a stable tertiary structure that covers the cell almost completely. These proteins bind to the cell wall non-covalently and could be partially detached on contacting the sorbent, which would disturb cell functioning and reproduction. One may also speculate that the hyper-crosslinked polystyrenes absorb certain blood constituent(s) which facilitate the growth of gram-positive bacteria but do not affect considerably the proliferation of gram-negative bacteria.

In addition, all sorbents examined were found to exert a pronounced influence on *S. cerevisiae* yeast suspended in canine blood by reducing their amount and decreasing the proportion of live fungi in the remaining fraction (by 82 % and 26 % for Styrosorb 514, 74 % and 27 % for carbon, and 76 % and 12 % for Styrosorb 514 M, respectively) (Figure 4.6) [71].

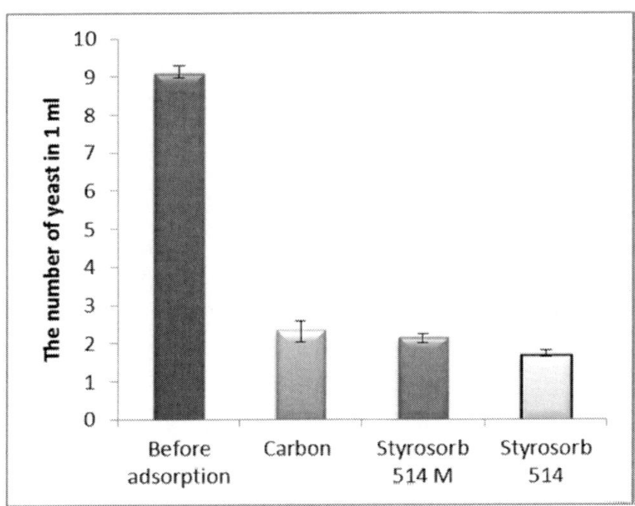

Figure 4.6. The number of yeast *S. cerevisiae* in spiked canine blood before and after contacting carbon hemosorbent Adsorba 300C, Styrosorb 514M and Styrosorb 514.

As was already repeatedly stressed, the most important characteristic of potential hemosorbents is their compatibility with blood. To evaluate the hemocompatibility of hypercrosslinked polystyrene Styrosorbs Anisimova et al. examined the hemolysis of erythrocytes, which is a consequence of cell membrane damage, as well as the destruction of mononuclear leukocytes (ML) in blood of healthy donors after blood's contact with the sorbents [71, 73]. Perfect hemocompatibility of Styrosorbs follows from Table 4.8 which lists results of the test. Indeed, within 4 hours of contact with the donor blood polymers cause only a minimal damage of erythrocytes. The same is true for the one hour-long incubation of ML suspension with the sorbents; the survival of leukocytes remains on a level of 90-99 %.

The obvious superiority in hemocompatibility of the polymers Styrosorb over granulated carbon hemosorbent becomes evident from the results of *in vitro* experiments with human blood. 10 mL of healthy donor blood stabilized with sodium citrate were recirculated 20 times through a miniature column with about 0.9 g sorbent at a flow rate of 1.3 mL/min. The averaged data are given in Figure 4.7.

After a 20-fold percolation of the human blood samples through Styrosorb 514, the hemolysis of erythrocytes and the aggregation of platelets did not exceed 5 %, thus demonstrating an excellent hemocompatibility of the polymer. Another hypercrosslinked sorbent, composite material Styrosorb 514M, under the same conditions also exhibits good hemocompatibility though, still, it is inferior a little to Styrosorb 514. Activated carbon-type hemosorbent, on the contrary, demonstrates an unsatisfactory performance.

Hypercrosslinked sorbents can also be used for the extracorporeal detoxification of lymphatic fluid [71]. This conclusion was drawn after percolating 700 mL lymph of an oncology patient in sepsis through a 80 mL column packed with Styrosorb 514. The comparison of biochemical and immunological lymph parameters before and after sorption procedure documented an insignificant lowering of total proteins concentration and practically invariable albumin concentration. It is quite interesting that Styrosorb 514 extracts 20 % urea and 39 % creatinine and reduces the concentration of LPS endotoxin by a factor of 7.4. At the same time the level of the lipopolysaccharide-binding protein (LBP) rises by a factor of 1.34. The latter fact appears to be caused by the destruction of LPS-LBP complex, followed by the sorption of LPS. In addition, the hypercrosslinked polystyrene sorbent decreased the concentration of pro-inflammatory cytokines IL-6, IL-18 and IL-8 by a factor of 1.6, 1.6 and 2.4, respectively.

Table 4.8. Hemolytic activity and toxicity for mononuclear leucocytes of hypercrosslinked polystyrenes measured after their contact with healthy donor blood (simple average and "min÷max" values)

Sorbent	ML survival rate, %	Hemolysis of erythrocytes, %		
		Time of incubation, hours		
		2	4	24
Styrosorb 516	**87**	**0**	**0**	**22**
	81÷91	*0÷5,5*	*0÷6,1*	*19,1÷28,9*
Styrosorb 514	**93**	**3**	**5**	**12**
	91÷100	*1,3÷10,5*	*1,7÷7,1*	*11,2÷14,7*
Styrosorb 414	**99**	**0**	**0**	**4**
	91÷100	*0÷4,8*	*0÷4,3*	*3,1÷4,0*

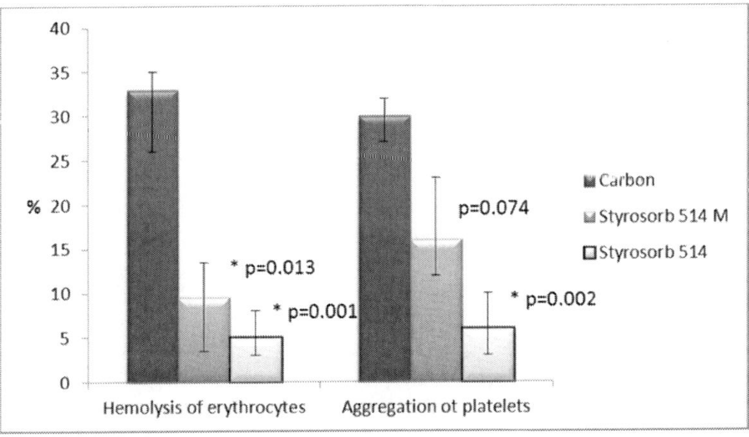

Figure 4.7. Hemolysis of erythrocytes and aggregation of platelets, % of initial, after recirculation of human blood through hypercrosslinked polystyrene sorbents and activated carbon hemosorbent Adsorba 300C [71].

In view of all the above findings, it was pretty safe to start conducting *in vivo* experiments on rabbits, aimed at the detoxification of blood at an early stage of an artificial septic shock [74, 75]. A group of 6 rabbits received under narcosis a portion of heparin (50 U/kg) and an intravenous infusion of 5 ng/kg lipopolysaccharide LPS *Klebsiella pneumoniae* (Sigma, USA) and 1000 U/kg recombinant human TNFв (Biosourse, USA). Blood circulation at a rate of 4 ml/min through a 10 ml column with Styrosorb 514 was organized using a peristaltic pump and a tubing line between the carotid artery and the jugular vein of the animal. Blood samples were taken from auricular veins before the experiment, three minutes after the injection of toxins and 1 hour afterwards. Three rabbits received hemoperfusion treatment during this 1 hour period while three other animals were left as the reference group.

Both the LPS and hTNFв cytokine appeared in the venous blood of rabbits already three minutes after injection. But, LPS was almost completely eliminated from blood of experimental animals within the 1 hour hemoperfusion treatment, while in the reference group it dropped to the half of the initial level (p=0.017), only. Similarly, concentration of hTNFв was reduced in the blood of animals under hemoperfusion 2.3 times stronger as in the reference group. Thus, hemoperfusion was found to efficiently eliminate bacterial LPS (to nearly 100 %) and pro-inflammatory cytokine TNFв (to over 60 %) at the early stage of the beginning acute systemic inflammatory process. Indeed, in the reference group of animals this process clearly manifested itself by a substantial drop in the neutrophils count and a rise in the leucocytes count, while no change in leucocytes and no hemolysis was registered in the group of animals that received hemoperfusion almost immediately after poisoning.

The above presented results of intensive *in vitro* and *in vitro* examination of tree different samples of hypercrosslinked polystyrene-type sorbents, Styrosorbs 514, 516 and 414, as well as composite material Styrosorb 514M on the base of an analogous polymer, all specially prepared for hemoperfusion tests, unambiguously prove their suitability for a practical application in the capacity of hemosorbents. By considering the whole complex of most important properties, all of them outperform the commercially available surface modified activated carbon-type hemosorbent Adsorba 300C. Styrosorb 514 was rated the best of the four hypercrosslinked polymeric samples under examination. While being mechanically stable and fully hemocompatible, it must exert a complex action on sepsis patients, simultaneously removing from blood circulation bacterial lipopolysaccharide-type endotoxins, numerous cytokines, pro- and anti-inflammatory factors and other middle-sized toxic proteins, as well as blocking proliferation of gram-positive bacteria and even fungi.

CONCLUSION

When summarizing all the data presented in this Chapter, we have every reason to conclude that the hypercrosslinked polystyrene-type sorbent Styrosorb 514, just like the earlier developed with our participation hypercrosslinked polydivinylbenzene-type BetaSorb™ and CytoSorb™, have several serious advantages over the currently applied modified activated carbon-type hemosorbents like Adsorba 300C. First of all, all hypercrosslinked polymeric sorbents exhibit an unprecedented hemocompatibility. Thus, Styrosorb 514 does not cause any damage of erythrocytes, a decrease in leukocyte count and aggregation of platelets. Styrosorb 514 eliminates almost completely the bacterial endotoxin LPS from blood of patients and significantly decreases concentration of most cytokines and excessive inflammatory factors. Importantly, Styrosorb 514 sorbent was found to eliminate a significant portion of low-molecular-weight toxic organic compounds, as well as urea, bilirubin and creatinine. Quite interesting is the fact that the sorbent suppresses propagation of toxic gram-positive bacteria and monocellular yeast fungi *S. cerevisiae*. In all cases the hemoperfusion through Styrosorb 514 provides much deeper blood detoxification than activated carbons do.

Now we have every reason to state that the hypercrosslinked polystyrene-type materials present very promising hemosorbents which can render a rapid and indispensable assistance in treating sepses patients. Moreover, it can also be considered a basic means of taking care in intensive therapy of most acute intoxications and inflammatory problems, including pneumonia and even avian influenza. The extremely high mortality, 61 % according to World Health Organization for the avian influenza epidemic of 2007, is a consequence of an overactive inflammatory response due to the virus-induced cytokine deregulation [76].

Following the remarkably successful use of Styrosorb 514 in the practice of veterinary clinics (see next Chapter), at the present day the material passed all official clinical tests and will soon appear in a regular use in Russian hospitals.

REFERENCES

[1]   Muirhead, EE; Reid, AF. *J. Lab. Clin. Med.*, 1948, 33, 841 – 844.

[2]   Yatzidis, H. *Proc. Eur. Dial. Transplant. Assos.*, 1964, 1, 83 – 86.

[3]   Gejyo, F; Yamada, T; Odani, S; Nakagava, Y; Arakawa, M; Kunitomo, T; Kataoka, H; Suzuki, M; Hirasawa, Y; Shirahama, T; Cohen, AS; Schmid, K. *Biochem. Biophys. Res. Commun.*, 1985, 129, 701 – 706.

[4]   Odell, RA; Slowiaczek, P; Moran, JE; Schindhelm, K. *Kidney Int.*, 1991, 39, 909 – 919.

[5]   Leypoldt, JK; Cheung, AK; Deeter, RB. *Am. J. Kidney Ass.*, 1998, 32, 295 – 301.

[6]   Klinke, B; Rockel, A; Abdelhamid, S; Fiegel, P; Walb, D. *Int. J. Artif. Organs*, 1989. 12, 697 – 702.

[7]   Ronco, C; Heifetz, A; Fox, K; Curtin, C; Brendolan, A; Gastaldon, P; Crepaldi, C; Fortunato, A; Pietribasi, G; Carbelotto, A; Brunello, A; Manami, SM; Zanella, M; La Greca, G. *Int. J. Artif. Organs*, 1997. 20, 136 – 143.

[8]   Winchester, JF; Ronco, C. *Adv. Renal Replacement Therapy*, 2002. 9, 19 – 25.

[9]   Chang, TMS. *Trans. Am. Soc. Artif. Intern. Organs*, 1966. 12, 13 – 19.

[10]   Kokot, F; Pietrek, J; Seredynski, M. *Proc. Eur. Dial. Transplant. Assos.*, 1978. 15, 604 – 606.

[11]   Winchester, JF. *Hemoperfusion in Replacement of Renal Function by Dialysis.* 3rd Edition. Dordrecht: Kluwer Academic; 1988, 439 – 459.

[12]   Furuyoshi, S; Kobayashi, A; Tamai, N; Yasuda, A; Tanaka, S; Tani, N; Nakazawa, R; Mimura, H; Gejyo, F; Arakawa, M. *Blood Purif.*, 1991, 9, 9.

[13]   Gejyo, F; Teramura, T; Ei I; Arakawa, M; Nakazawa, T. *Artif. Organs*, 1995, 19, 1222 – 1226.

[14]   Miyata, T; Jadoul, M; Kurokawa, K; Van Ypersele de Strihou, C. *J. Am. Soc. Nephrol.*, 1998, 9, 1723 – 1735.

[15]   Davankov, VA; Tsyurupa, MP; Pavlova, LA; Tur, DR. *Bio- and hemocompatible sorbents based on hypercrosslinked styrene polymers with modified surface, methods of obtaining the same and method of obtaining the sorbent matrix*, Patent RF 2.089.283, 1997.

[16]   Davankov, VA; Tsyurupa, MP; Pavlova, LA; Tur, DR. *Sorbents for removing toxicants from blood or plasma, and method of producing the same*, Patent USA 5.773.384, 1998.

[17]   Rogozhin, SV; Davankov, VA; Tsyurupa, MP. *Method of obtaining macronet styrene copolymers*, Patent USSR 299165, 1969; Patents: USA 3,729,457, Austria 312929, Australia 448487, Great Britain 1315214, Argentina 190867, Belgium 756082, DDR 85644, Holland 140869, Canada 909442, Italy 916194, France 2061341, FRG 2045096, Czechoslovakia 164371, Switzerland 542254, Japan 982759; C.A., 75 (1971) 6841b.

[18]   Davankov, VA; Tsyurupa, MP. In: Aharoni S, editor. *Synthesis, Characterization and Theory of Polymeric Networks and Gels.* Plenum Press, 1992, 179 – 200.

[19] Strom, RM; Murray, DJ. *Device for removing toxins from blood or plasma*, Patent USA, 6, 419, 830, 2002.

[20] Strom, RM; Murray, DJ. *Surface modified polymer beads*, Patent USA 6, 338, 801, 2002.

[21] Strom, RM; Murray, DJ. *Surface modified polymer beads*, Patent USA 6, 238, 795, 2001.

[22] Strom, RM; Murray, DJ. *Device for removing toxins from blood or plasma*, Patent USA 6, 423, 024, 2002.

[23] Young, W-T; Albright, RL. *Size-selective hemoperfusion polymeric adsorbents*, Patent USA 7, 875, 182, 2011.

[24] Davankov, VA; Tsyurupa, MP; Pavlova, LA. *Method of making biocompatible polymeric adsorbing material for purification of physiological fluids of organism*, Patent USA 6, 531, 523, 2003.

[25] Nanko, T; Furuyoshi, S; Takata, S; Nakatani, M. *Adsorbent and method for adsorbing a chemokine in body fluid*, Patent USA 7, 279, 106, 2007.

[26] Nanko, T; Furuyoshi, S; Takata, S; Nakatani, M. *Device for body fluid purification and system for body fluid purification*, Patent USA 6, 878, 269, 2005.

[27] Brady, JA; Winchester, JF; Davankov, VA; Tsyurupa, MP; Pavlova, LA; Quartararo, PJ; Salsberg, JA. *Devices, systems, and methods for reducing levels of pro-inflammatory or anti-inflammatory stimulators or mediators in the blood*, Patent USA 6, 878, 127, 2005.

[28] Brady, JA; Winchester, JF; Davankov, V; Tsyurupa, M; Pavlova, L; Norris, F; Quartararo, PJ; Salsberg, JA. *Devices, systems, and methods for reducing levels of pro-inflammatory or anti-inflammatory stimulators or mediators in the blood, generated as a result of extracorporeal blood processing*, Patent USA 7, 312, 023, 2007.

[29] Brady, JA; Winchester, JF; Davankov, VA; Tsyurupa, MP; Pavlova, LA; Noris, FM; Quartararo PJ; Salsberg JA. *Biocompatible devices, systems, and methods for reducing levels of pro-inflammatory or anti-inflammatory stimulators or mediators in the blood*, Patent USA 7 7, 556, 768, 2009.

[30] Brady, JA; Winchester, JF; Davankov, VA; Tsyurupa, MP; Pavlova, LA; Noris, FM. *Methods for reducing levels of pro-inflammatory or anti-inflammatory stimulators or mediators in the blood*, Patent USA 7, 846, 650, 2010.

[31] Hei, DJ. *Adsorbing pathogen-inactivating compounds with porous particles immobilized in a matrix*, Patent USA 7, 611, 831, 2009.

[32] Hei, DJ. Removing compounds from blood products with porous particles immobilized in a matrix, Patent USA 7, 037, 642, 2007.

[33] Hei, DJ. *Absorbing pathogen-inactivating compounds with porous particles immobilized in a matrix*, Patent USA 6, 951, 713, 2005.

[34] Hei, DJ. *Methods and devices for the removal of psoralens from blood products,* Patent USA 6, 544, 727, 2003.

[35] Nakamura, K. Komiya, K; Fujii, S. *Process for production of partially hydrophilized porous adsorbents*, Patent USA 6, 900, 157, 2005.

[36] Matson, JR. *Hemofiltration systems, methods and devices for treatment of chronic and acute diseases*, Patent USA 7, 758, 533, 2010.

[37] Matson JR. *Hemofiltration methods for treatment of diseases in a mammal*, Patent USA 7, 291, 122, 2007.

[38] Hughes, RD. Review of methods to remove protein-bound substances in liver failure. *Int. J. Artif. Organs*, 2002 25, 911 - 977.

[39] Roberts, CP; Litzie, K. *Plasma detoxification and volume control system and methods of use*, Patent USA 8, 038, 638, 2011.

[40] Weber, V; Linsberger, I; Hauner, M; Leistner, A; Leistner, A; Falkenhagen, D. Neutral styrene divinylbenzene copolymers for adsorption of toxins in liver failure. *Biomacromolecules*, 2008 9, 1322 – 1328.

[41] Eichhorn, T; Ivanov, AE; Dainiak, MB; Leistner, A; Linsberger, I; Jungvid, H; Mikhalovsky, SV; Weber, V; Macroporous Composite Cryogels with Embedded Polystyrene Divinylbenzene Microparticles for the Adsorption of Toxic Metabolites from Blood. *Journal of Chemistry*, 2013, Article ID 348412, 8 pages, http://dx.doi.org/10.1155/2013/ 348412.

[42] Falkenhagen, D; Brandl, M; Hartmann, J; Kellner, KH; Posnicek, T; Weber, V. Fluidized bed adsorbent systems for extracorporeal liver support. *Therapeutic Apheresis and Dialysis*, 2006 10, 154 – 159.

[43] Leistner, A; Leistner, A. *Adsorbing material for blood and plasma cleaning method and for albumin purification*, European Patent EP1578526, 2005, Patent USA 7, 311, 845, 2007.

[44] Eguchi, T; Tsunomori, M. *Method of making uniform polymer particles*, Patent USA 5, 015, 425, 1991.

[45] Sherman, JD; Bem, DJ. *Process for removing toxins from blood using zirconium metallate or titanium metallate compositions*, Patent USA 6, 099, 737, 2000.

[46] Sherman, JD. *Process for removing toxins from bodily fluids using zirconium or titanium microporous compositions*, Patent USA 6, 332, 985, 2001.

[47] Davankov, VA; Rogozhin, SV; Tsyurupa, MP. Patent USSR 299165 (1969); Chem. Abstr., 75 (1971) 6841b; Patent USA 3, 729, 457.

[48] Davankov, VA; Tsyurupa, MP. Hypercrosslinked Polymeric Networks and Adsorbing Materials. Synthesis, Structure, Properties, and Application. *Comprehensive Analytical Chemistry.* Elsevier; 2011, 56; 670 p.

[49] Tsyurupa, MP; Davankov, VA. *Reactive & Functional Polymers*, 2002, 53, 193 – 203.

[50] Davankov, VA; Elizarov, DP; El'kin, AI; Kataev, SS; Pavlova, KA; Terekhin, GA; Tsyurupa, MP. *Toxicological Bulletin* (Russia), 2002, 3, 2 – 5.

[51] Elizarov, DP; El'kin, AI; Davankov, VA; Kataev, SS; Pavlova, LA; Reshetnikov, VI; Terekhin, GA; Tsyurupa, MP. *Efferent therapy* (Russia), 2003, 9, 58 – 61.

[52] Elizarov, DP; El'kin, AI; Davankov, VA; Kataev, SS; Pavlova, LA; Reshetnikov, VI; Terekhin, GA; Tsyurupa, MP. *Toxicological Bulletin* (Russia), 2003, 2, 18 – 21.

[53] Davankov, V; Pavlova, L; Tsyurup, M; Brady, J; Balsamo, M; Yousha. E. *J. Chromatogr. B*, 2000 739, 73 – 80.

[54] Malik, DJ; Webb, C; Holdich, RG; Ramsden, JJ; Warwick, GL; Roche, I; Williams, DJ; Trochimzcuk, AW; Dale, JA; Hoenich, NA. *Separation and Purification Technology*, 2009, 66, 578 – 585.

[55] Beth, M; Unger, KK; Tsyurupa, MP; Davankov, VA. *Chromatographia*, 1993, 36, 351 – 355.

[56] Ronco, C; Heifetz, A; Fox, K; Curtin, C; Brendolan, A; Gastaldon, P; Crepaldi, C; Fortunato, A; Pietribasi, G; Carbelotto, A; Brunello, A; Manami, SM; Zanella, M; La Greca, G. *Int. J. Artif. Organs*, 1997, 20, 136 – 143.

[57] Bosh T; Wendler T; Duhr C; Brady J; Samtleben W. *J. Am. Soc. Nephrol.*, 2000, 11, 257A.

[58] Ronco, C; Brendolan, A; Winchester, JF; Golds, E; Clemmer, J; Polaschegg, HD; Muller, TE; La Greca, G; Levin, NW. *Blood Purif.*, 2001, 19, 260 – 263.

[59] Winchester, JF; Ronco, C; Brady, JA; Cowgill, LD; Salsberg, J; Yousha, E; Choquette, M; Albright, R; Clemmer, J; Davankov, V; Tsyurupa, M; Pavlova, L; Pavlov, M; Cohen, G; Hurl, W; Gotch, F; Levin, NW. The next step from high flux dialysis: Application of sorbent technology. *Blood Purif.*, 2002, 20, 81 - 86.

[60] Winchester, JF; Ronco, C; Brady, JA; Golds, E; Clemmer, J; Cowgill, LD; Muller, TE; Levin, NW. *Blood Purif.*, 2001, 19, 255 – 259.

[61] Morena, MD; Guo, D; Balakrishnan, VS; Brady, JA; Winchester, JF; Jaber, BL. *Kidney Intern.*, 2003, 63, 1150 – 1154.

[62] Winchester, JF; Kellum, JA; Ronco, C; Brady, JA; Quartararo, P; Salsberg, J; Levin, NW; Sorbents in acute renal failure and the systemic inflammatory response syndrome. *Blood Purif.*, 2003, 21, 79 - 84.

[63] Winchester, JF; Ronco, C. Sorbent Hemoperfusion in End Stage Renal Disease: An In-Depth Review. *Advances in Renal Replacement Therapy*, 2002, 9, 19 - 25.

[64] Kellum, JA; Song, M; Venkataraman, R; Hemoadsorption removes tumor necrosis factor, interleukin-6, and interleukin-10, reduces nuclear factor - kappa-B DNA binding, and improves short-term survival in lethal endotoxemia. *Critical Care Medicine*, 2004, 32, 801 – 805.

[65] Peng, ZY; Carter, MJ; Kellum, JA; Effect of hemoadsorption on cytokine removal and short-term survival in septic rats. *Critical Care Medicine*, 2008, 36, 1573-1577.

[66] Tetta, C; Bellomo, R; Inquaqqiato; Wratten, ML; Ronco, C. Endotoxin and cytokine removal in sepsis. *Ther. Apher.* 2002, 6(2), 109 – 115.

[67] Brady, JA; Winchester, JF; Davankov, VA; Tsvurupa, MP; Pavlova, LA; Norris, FM; Quartararo, Jr PJ; Salsberg, JA. *Methods for reducing levels of pro-inflammatory or anti-inflammatory stimulators or mediators in the blood*, Patent USA 8, 349, 550, 2013.

[68] www.cytosorbents.com

[69] Anisimova, NYu; Dolzhikova, YuI; Davankov, VA; Pastukhov, AV; Miljaeva, SI; Senatov, FS; Kiselevsky, MV. Prospects for the application of biporous sorbents based on hypercrosslinked styrene polymers for the prevention and treatment of systemic purulent-septic complications. *Nanotechnologies in Russia*, 2012, 7 № 5–6, 318–326.

[70] Malika, DJ; Warwick, GL; Venturi, M; Streat, M; Hellgardt, K; Hoenich, N; Dale, JA. Preparation of novel mesoporous carbons for the adsorption of an inflammatory cytokine (IL-1b). *Biomaterials,* 2004, 25, 2933 – 2940.

[71] Anisimova, NYu. Pathogenetic reasons for use of extracorporeal detoxification of cancer patients with sepsis. *Dr. Sci. Thesis*, Moscow; 2012.

[72] Anisimova, NYu; Davankov, VA; Budnik, MI; Spirina, TS; Kiselevsky, MV. New perspective sorbents based on polystyrene, capable of eliminating microorganisms from blood. *Russian Journal of Biotherapy*, 2010, 9 № 4, 113 – 114.

[73] Anisimova, NYu; Dolzhikova, YuI; Davankov, VA; Pastukhov, AV; Miljaeva, SI; Senatov, FS; Kiselevsky, MV. Hemocompatibility of nanostructured sorbents based on hypercrosslinked styrene polymers of the Styrosorb series. *Russian Journal of Biotherapy*, 2012, 11 № 1, 23 – 29.

[74] Anisimova, NYu; Davankov, VA; Budnik, MI; Donenko, FV; Tuguz, AR; Kiselevsky, MV. Prospects of the use of nanoporous sorbent Stirosorb 514 for extracorporeal detoxification at system inflammatory reaction and sepsis. *Vestnik of Adyghe State University* (Russian), 2011, 1(76), 91 – 98.

[75] Anisimova, NYu; Davankov, VA; Kornyushenkov, EA; Mitin, VV; Solov'eva, OV; Budnik, MI; Donenko, FV; Kiselevsky, MV. Efficacy of hypercrosslinked polystyrene for extracorporeal detoxification in the animals with endotoxin shock. *Russian Veterinary Journal* (Russian), 2011, 2, 23 – 25.

[76] Us, D. Cytokine storm in avian influenza (Review). *Microbiol. Bul.*, 2008, 42, 365-380.

In: Immunological Pathogenesis of Sepsis ...   ISBN: 978-1-62948-674-1
Editor: Natalia Yu. Anisimova   © 2014 Nova Science Publishers, Inc.

Chapter 5

AN EXPERIENCE OF APPLICATION OF THE DEVICE BASED ON THE HEMOSORBENT STYROSORB 514 IN TREATMENT OF DOGS WITH SEPSIS (PILOT STUDY)

N. Yu. Anisimova[1], V. A. Davankov[2],*
M. P. Tsyurupa[2], L. A. Pavlova[2], E. A. Kornjushenkov[1],
E. V. Zakharov[1], N. V. Ustyuzhanina[3]
and M. V. Kiselevsky[1]

[1]N.N. Blokhin Russian Cancer Research Center, Russian Academy of Medical Sciences, Moscow, Russian Federation
[2]A.N. *Nesmeyanov Institute of Organoelement Compounds*, Russian Academy of Sciences, Moscow, Russian Federation
[3]N.D. Zelinsky Institute of Organic Chemistry, Russian Academy of Sciences, Moscow, Russian Federation

ABSTRACT

This chapter describes the results of a pilot study on the use of the experimental device based on polystyrene sorbent Styrosorb 514 for the treatment of 5 dogs with sepsis.

---

* n.yu.anisimova@gmail.com.

Exceptional hemocompatibility and sorption properties of the hypercrosslinked polystyrene-type sorbents of Styrosorb series, now documented beyond all doubts, permitted practical implementation of Styrosorb 514 in hemoperfusion studies *in vivo*.

Dogs with cancer and with symptoms of multiple organ failure that accompanies sepsis were chosen for the study. The animals were divided into 2 groups, 5 dogs in each. Hemosorption was carried out on "Hemos-HS" (Biotech-M, Russia) apparatus, basically consisting of a special peristaltic pump coupled with one of two types of columns (100 mL). "Hemos-KS" (Biotech-M, Russia) based on carbon sorbent was used for hemoperfusion in the control group of animals, while a glass column packed with Styrosorb 514 was used for the experimental animal group (Figure 5.1). Heparin load was 100-200 U/kg and the time of hemoperfusion treatment was 2 h. Thus, the volume of sorbents, the period of treatment, hardware, and pharmaceutical support of the patients were similar in the both groups.

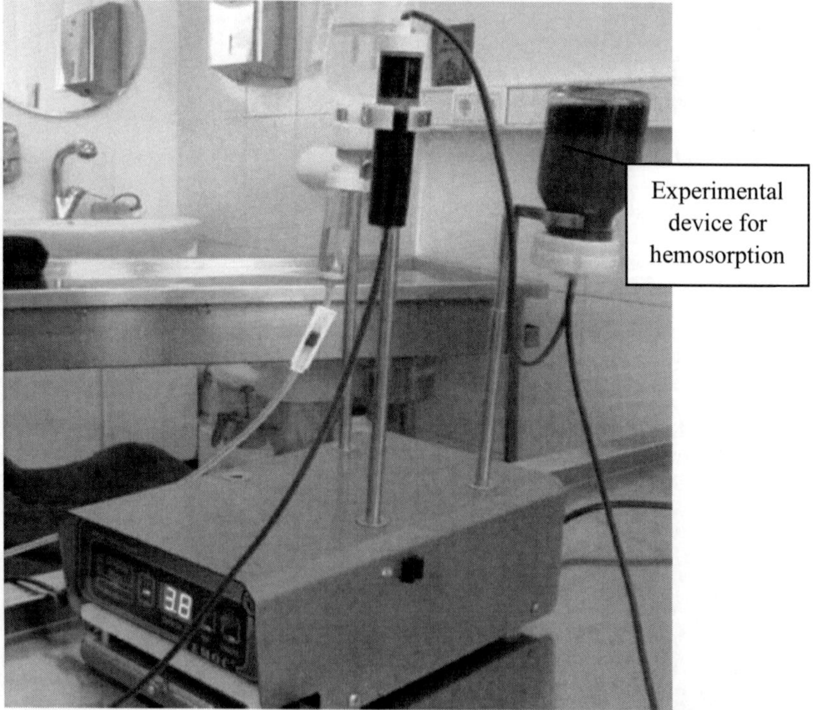

Figure 5.1. The extracorporeal hemosorption with experimental device based on Styrosorb 514.

Venous blood sampling was performed before, 3 minutes after hemosorption, as well as 24 hours after the treatment (points 1, 2 and 3, correspondingly). In these three reference points, the physiological state of the animals (cardiovascular system parameters and cognitive functions) was estimated, and instrumental analysis of biochemical, hematological and immunological parameters of the blood were performed for the animals in the both groups.

Significant improvement of general clinical state and cognitive functions (motor activity of the animals and their response to external irritants), as well as normalization of cardiovascular function (increasing of initially low systolic arterial pressure (AP) by $21\pm2.1\%$ and mean AP by $24\pm1.4\%$, $p<0.05$) were observed for the animals after hemoperfusion using hypercrosslinked polystyrene column. Moreover, as opposed to the control animals, the treatment in experimental group didn't cause any changes of pH and ionic composition of blood serum, as well as didn't lead to decreasing of erythrocytes and platelets concentrations in system blood flow. Obviously, the last observation indicated the absence of platelet aggregation, which implies relative tolerance of blood coagulation factors to the contact with the polymer sorbent.

As stimulation of blood coagulation is known to be one of the major negative effects of carbon-type sorbents application for extracorporeal detoxification, this aspect was examined especially thorough during the clinical study. According to the data obtained, neither significant signs of bleeding, nor increasing of blood coagulation tendency were observed during and after hemoperfusion through the experimental hypercrosslinked polystyrene column.

Notably, changes in blood levels of metabolites, bacterial endotoxin (LPS) and albumin were observed in the both groups of animals after hemosorption (Table 5.1).

In comparison with carbon sorbent, Styrosorb 514 was found to provide substantially more effective elimination of several toxic metabolites from animal blood, such as urea (59 %), creatinine (30 %), bilirubin (77 %, $p = 0.007$), and LPS (100 %, $p = 0.031$), while no depletion of albumin concentration was observed. Moreover, a significant decrease in serum concentrations of the above toxic metabolites 24 hours after hemosorption was established only in the case of the experimental column with the polystyrene sorbent. These facts indicate attenuation of the inflammation in pancreas and liver of treated patients, which could be considered as a positive system response of the organism to the hemosorption treatment, particularly, to the elimination of triggers of inflammation. In fact, the both columns were shown to bind bacterial LPS effectively (81-100 %), however the application of the experimental polymeric column demonstrated more prolonged detoxification effect (Figure 5.2).

Table 5.1. Changes of blood levels of metabolites, bacterial endotoxin (LPS) and albumin after HS in dogs with sepsis

Analytes	Hemosorbent	Before hemosorption*	After hemosorption*	Norma for healthy dogs
Urea, mmol/L	Styrosorb 514	19 *(11-22)*	7.8 *(7-16)*	*3.5-10.0*
	Carbon	15 *(8-38)*	10 *(6-34)*	
Creatinine, μmol/L	Styrosorb 514	148 *(92-203)*	104 *(102-224)*	*45-140*
	Carbon	152 *(89-363)*	132 *(101-303)*	
Bilirubin, μmol/L	Styrosorb 514	53 *(30-76)*	12** *(9-15)*	*0-12*
	Carbon	23 *(6-66)*	29 *(8-71)*	
LPS,U/mL	Styrosorb 514	0.114 *(0.097-0.241)*	0** *(0-0.003)*	*0-0.0001****
	Carbon	0.100 *(0.054-0.394)*	0.005 *(0-0.084)*	
Albumin, g/L	Styrosorb 514	28 *(27-29)*	30 *(24-36)*	*25-391*
	Carbon	31 *(19-43)*	22** *(20-24)*	

* Median *(25%-75%)*.

** $p < 0.05$.

*** –the results of own studies on healthy dogs (n=24).

Thereby, the advantages of the experimental column with the polymeric sorbent Styrosorb 514 in comparison with the previously used column based on modified carbon sorbent were demonstrated. The hemoperfusion device with the new sorbent could be effectively used in supply and correctional therapy in cases of selected organ failure (renal and hepatic failure, pancreatitis, etc.) and multiple organ failure. Besides, it could be used as a tool for detoxification in cases of LPS-mediated sepsis.

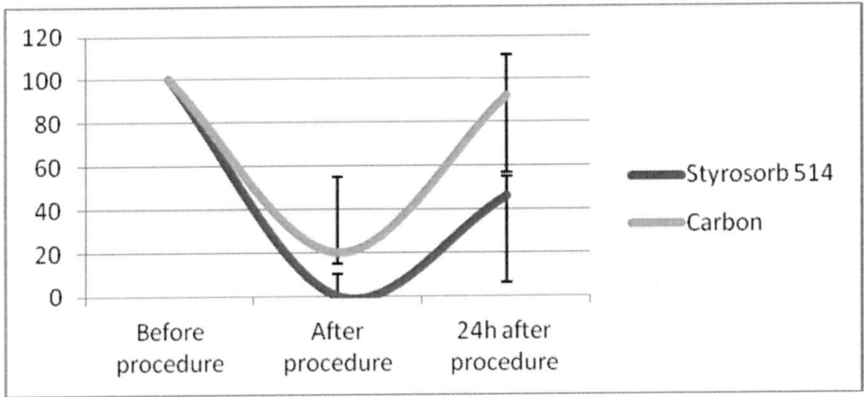

Figure 5.2. Change of LPS levels in the blood of dogs with sepsis after extracorporeal detoxification with the device based on Styrosorb 514 or carbon hemosorbents.

CONCLUSION

Overall, the results of the *in vivo* study demonstrated the significant clinical effectiveness of hemoperfusion therapy application in cases of development of SIRS accompanied by organ failure. It was definitely confirmed, that protein and metabolic profile of blood normalized after the treatment, and detoxification (significant decrease of LPS concentration in the blood) and immunocorrection processes in the organism took place. During the hemosorption procedure, the homeostasis of the organism was observed to restore, in the blood-mediated manner, on levels of cells, tissue and organs. Importantly, neither significant changes in the blood coagulation system, nor a noticeable fluctuation of serum albumin content were observed. As a result, experimental animals demonstrated normalization of cardiovascular system parameters and required less vasopressor support.

The whole complex of results obtained thus far could be regarded as a solid base for implementation of the new effective sorbents of Styrosorb type and the simple and reliable device for extracorporeal detoxification in health care practice, particularly, in oncology.

CONCLUSION

The data of the prospective study of the peculiarities of cellular and humoral immunity of cancer patients with sepsis and septic shock represented in first chapters of the monograph demonstrated non-specific nature of the observed disorders. The tests indicated a relative informativity of study of wide range of serum cytokines for sepsis diagnostic. Only three cytokines (IL-6, IL-10 and IL-18) from 13 analyzed mediators were shown to be diagnostic markers of severe sepsis and septic shock, and two cytokines (IL-8 and IL-10) could be considered as prognosis parameters of patients in terms of 28-day mortality. A significant increase of sR IL-1 II in the blood of patients with sepsis was also regarded as a poor prognostic sign. In addition, it was found that the concentration of LPS, sR TNF I and sCD14 in the blood serum of patients with sepsis and septic shock was significantly higher than those of healthy donors, whereas there were observed no significant differences in studied parameters of cancer patients with sepsis and septic shock in comparison with patients without septic complications and healthy donors. Study of cytokine-induced activity of blood cells of cancer patients with septic complications and healthy donors in vitro revealed excessive spontaneous production of IL-8 in sepsis on the background of unreactivity to additional antigenic stimulation, increase of activity of NK and neutrophils after stimulation by latex granules, yeasts and bacteria. Significant disorders in the phenotype of immune blood cells of cancer patients with sepsis were revealed. In particular, a significant increasing of CD11b expression on the membranes of leukocytes was noted along with a decreasing of CD95 expression and on the background of neutrophilia and reduction of the ratio of CD4/CD8, which let us to consider these changes as markers of sepsis development. Moreover, taking into consideration the identified high correlation of normalization of clinical parameters and dynamics of LPS and blood serum cytokines of patients, the indicated laboratory parameters can be regarded as parameters of evaluation of patient's state changes after therapeutic intervention, including methods of extracorporeal detoxification. Therefore, the variety and intensity of immune disorders that observe in septic patients are considered to be significant pathogenetic part of sepsis development. Furthermore, it was found that the pathological changes of the internal organs of experimental animals on the background of the toxicity, induced by LPS are similar to diagnosed by pathological material study of cancer patients with MODS against sepsis - that indicate about possibly leading role of bacterial endotoxins in the development of pathological process. Thus, these data show that both triggers (micro-organisms and their toxins) and inflammatory mediators (IL-6, IL-10, IL-18) that secreted by immune cells play an important role in the pathogenesis of SIRS and sepsis and so the impact on the parts of the inflammation cascade should be regarded as an essential component of a complex approach to the treatment of septic complications.

Based on the research of the effectiveness of hemosorption as one of the systemic therapeutic treatment in cancer patients with sepsis, it was found that the use of LPS-selective and low-selective exposure devices with carbon sorbent could significantly reduce the concentration of bacterial LPS and wide spectrum of cytokines in the systemic circulation, as well as the normalization of immune effectors' functional activity. Thus, the obtained data suggest the validity of the application of hemosorption in the treatment of sepsis and septic shock in cancer patients, especially in the form of a course of consistently repetitive procedures.

A number of a new materials perspective for use as hemosorbents were characterized in the monograph. In particular, there are results of comparative studies of the physical and sorption characteristics of hypercrosslinked polystyrene sorbents Styrosorb and commercial modified activated carbon-type hemosorbent. Polystyrene sorbents were found to be more perspective regarding to binding a wide range of serum cytokines and exogenous trigger and mediator factors of inflammation (microorganisms and their toxins) in a physiological solution and damaging of blood cells by repeated contact during perfusion.

Further the effectiveness of the experimental column based on Styrosorb 514 for extracorporeal detoxification on animals was studied. It was found that the result of 1 hour duration of HS with the use of an experimental column was nearly complete elimination of exogenous biomolecules from the blood circulation, when it was tested on rabbits with reproduced model of LPS/h

TNF-induced shock, while there was not achieved a significant reduction in determined blood analytes in rabbits of the control group (intact). The results of studies of the effectiveness of hemo- and lymphoperfusion through the experimental column in vitro and in vivo on dogs with organ failure against sepsis were more efficient elimination of LPS, urea, creatinine, bilirubin from the blood serum in comparison with control carbon device on the background of relative tolerance of blood coagulation system to contact with a polystyrene sorbent. Clinical trials on animals with signs of organ failure on the back ground of SIRS showed that application of extracorporeal detoxification in complex therapy with the use of hemosorption column model based on Styrosorb 514 led to the normalization of metabolite, water-electrolyte and protein composition of the blood circulation. The procedure had detoxifying (removal of LPS from the blood and nitrogen-containing products of protein metabolism) and immune correlated effect on the body against the absence of marked changes in blood coagulation and serum concentration of albumin. As a result, there were observed a reduction of vasopressor support, normalization of cardiovascular system parameters and cognitive functions of sick animals. Thus, the obtained results may form the basis of introduction of new effective sorbents of Styrosorb series and devices for extracorporeal detoxification to the practice of public health and, in particular, oncology.

INDEX

E

E.coli, 101
eczema, 58
edema, 30, 31, 32, 35, 36, 42
effusion, 30, 32, 33, 37
egg, 90
electrolyte, 123
electron, 100
embolism, 27, 32, 59, 62
emigration, 10
emphysema, 42
encephalopathy, 29
endangered, 22
endocarditis, 27
endorphins, 67
endothelial cells, 28, 29
endothelium, 10, 12, 32
endotoxemia, 13, 42, 53, 112
endotoxins, 26, 40, 45, 51, 70, 106, 122
end-stage renal disease, 61, 91, 94
England, 19
environment, 95
epidemic, 107
epidemiology, 19
epithelia, 60
epithelial cells, 31, 35, 39, 42
epithelium, 12, 31, 32, 33, 35, 36, 42
equilibrium, 60, 71, 80
equipment, 61, 73
erythrocytes, 31, 36, 85, 104, 105, 107, 117
ESRD, 61, 94
ethanol, 92
ethyl acetate, 72
ethylene, 68, 78, 84, 85, 88
ethylene glycol, 68
etiology, 47
European Union, 58, 98
evidence, 3, 6, 8, 12, 14, 52, 92
exclusion, 89
excretion, 50
exotoxins, 2
expenditures, 95
exposure, 95, 122
external environment, 27

extraction, 54, 82, 92
extracts, 67, 92, 104
extrusion, 73

F

fat, 30
fat embolism, 30
fatty acids, 73
fever, 38, 92
fiber(s), 61, 69, 70
fiber membranes, 61
fibrillation, 60, 72, 85
fibrin, 31, 33, 38, 39
fibrinogen, 62, 72
fibrinolysis, 47
fibroblast proliferation, 42
fibroblasts, 33
fibrosis, 32
filtration, 50, 64
flora, 12
fluid, 61, 104, 109
force, 99
formation, 31, 32, 64, 70, 73, 74, 76, 78, 79, 81, 85, 87
fragments, 73, 80
France, 108
free radical copolymerization, 66, 76, 88
free radicals, 67
free volume, 80
freezing, 69
fungal infection, 27
fungi, 17, 58, 69, 103, 106, 107
furan, 73
fusion, 20, 86

G

gastrointestinal tract, 52
gel, 70, 78, 80
Germany, 97
glomerulus, 26, 36, 39
glucocorticoid, 21
glucose, 62

H

I

J

K

L

M

T

U